I0165557

The Mindful Table

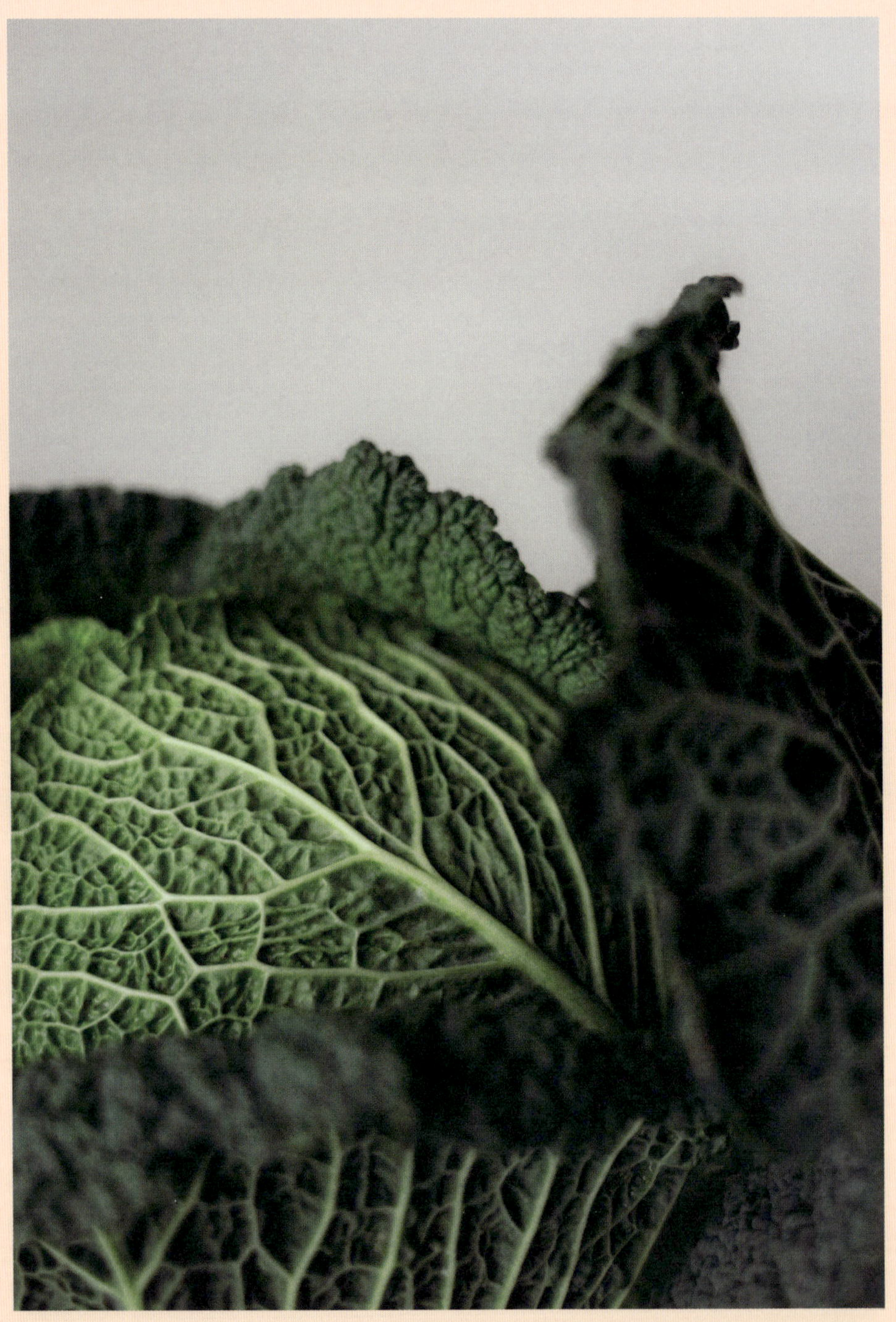

The Mindful Table

Recipes & Affirmations for Intuitive, Seasonal Eating

Cassandra Bodzak

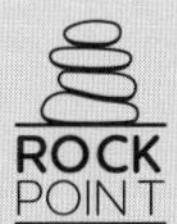

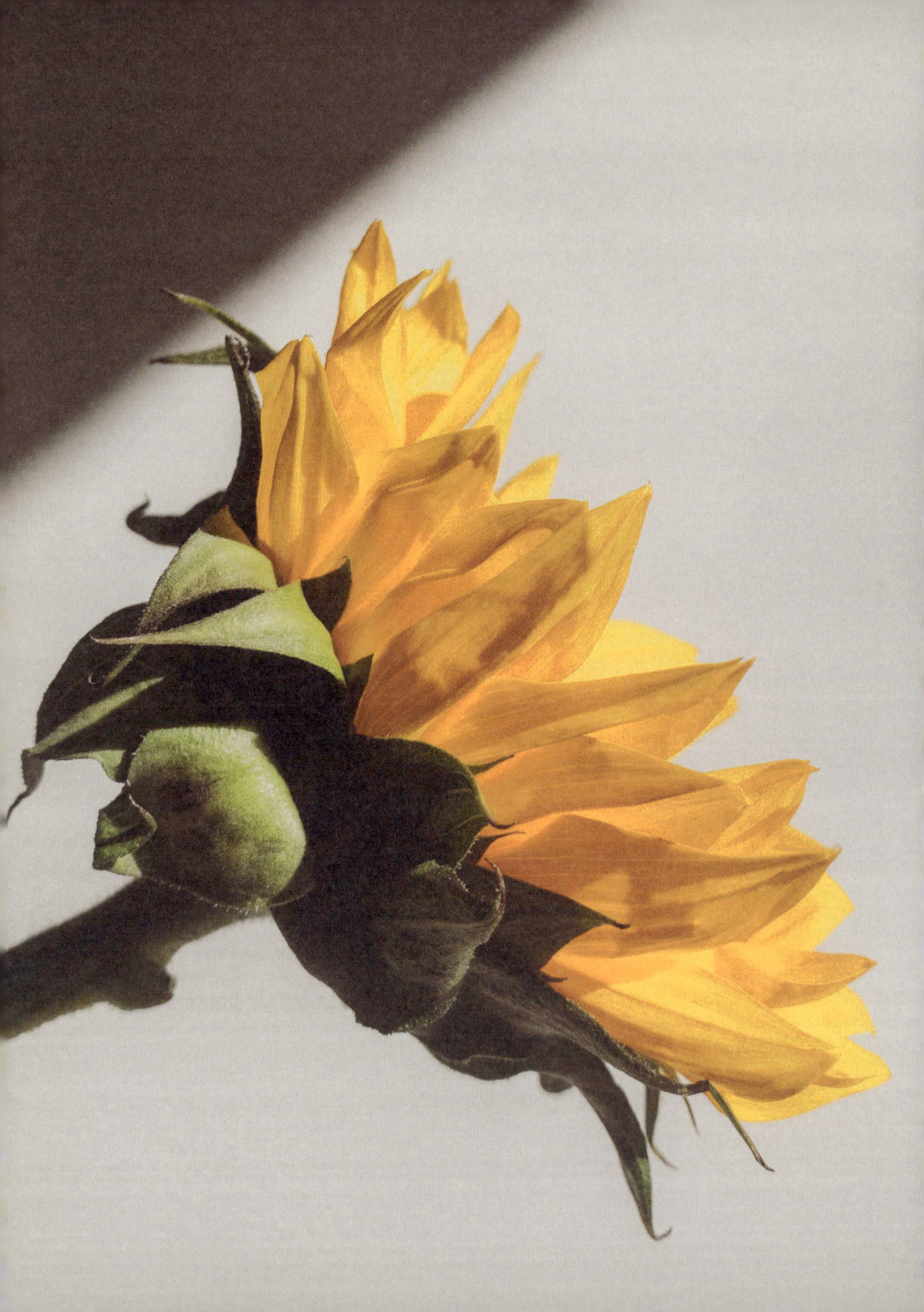

Contents

SUMMER

FALL

WINTER

INTRODUCTION
A Life That Lights You Up

This book is something that was birthed straight out of my soul. At its core, the book merges food, meditation, and self-care, teaching them all as one holistic system. Food, meditation, and self-care come together to help create a foundation that will support our most joyful lives on this planet. Each one is sacred and powerful on its own, but together they are unstoppable.

Food is one of those things that you can't escape. It's a necessity that can either work for you or against you. Ultimately, you have to decide if you want to take that relationship you have with food and your body to a more loving level. Your willingness to shift is the first domino that starts it all! People often don't even make it to the self-awareness stage if they are still trapped in the conversation around food and their body. However, when you break through, you'll see how meditation and self-care are potent tools that can really harness and elevate the powerful instruments that our minds and bodies are.

Through this first doorway of food, you will embark on a holistic journey of well-being and begin a life in which feeling good isn't an occasional occurrence, but an everyday gift. It is possible to eat amazing food that is healthy, makes you feel good, and puts you into a different energetic state, but the reality is that the food conversation is just the beginning. It's an entry point to a conversation that involves utilizing your mind, body, and soul to live your greatest life on Earth. It's not just about Instagram-ready smoothie bowls, vegan brownies, eating massive salads, and drinking green juice every day. It's about the intention behind it and your relationship with food. It's about the why. *Why are you eating this way?* I spent many years eating salads and drinking green juices from a really unhealthy place. I truly believe it would have been better for me to be eating french fries from a really loving place than eating the salads from a place of guilt and self-loathing.

In fact, let me say this now: I don't care if you use the recipes in this book. I hope they simply get you in the kitchen and in the joy of nourishing yourself. It's about shifting the conversation you have every single day about what you are putting on your plate; it's about getting you into a loving and nurturing relationship with your body; and it's about creating rituals in your life by incorporating meditation and simple self-care exercises so that you can be fully supported in living your best life with a clear head, open heart, and boundless energy.

We are all at different points in our food-life journey, and I wish I'd had this book as a guide when I first started out. I look forward to walking beside you on your journey to eating with intention and showing you the blueprint to designing a life that lights you up from the inside out. Trust me, if it was possible for me, I know it's possible for you too!

Cassandra Bodzak

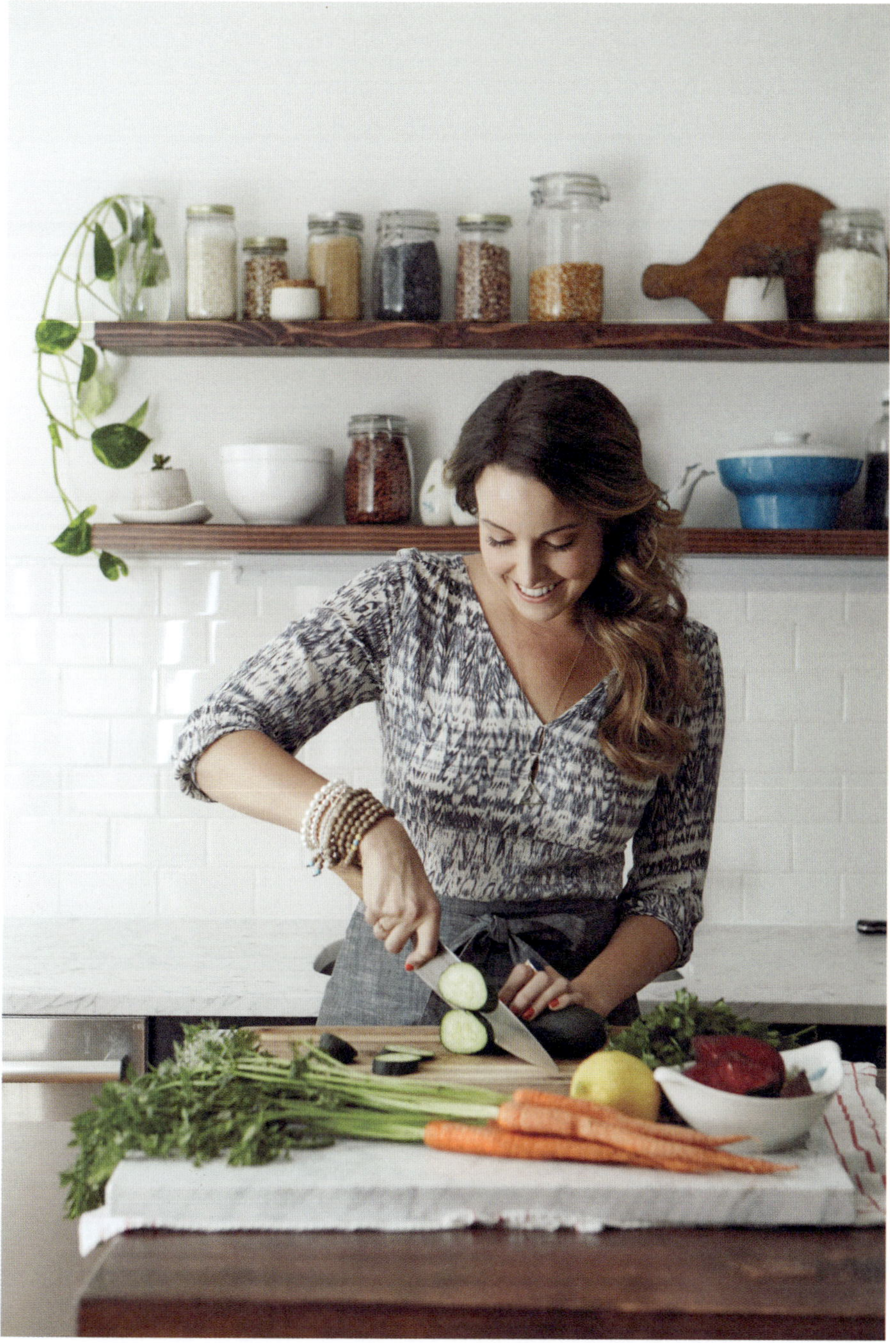

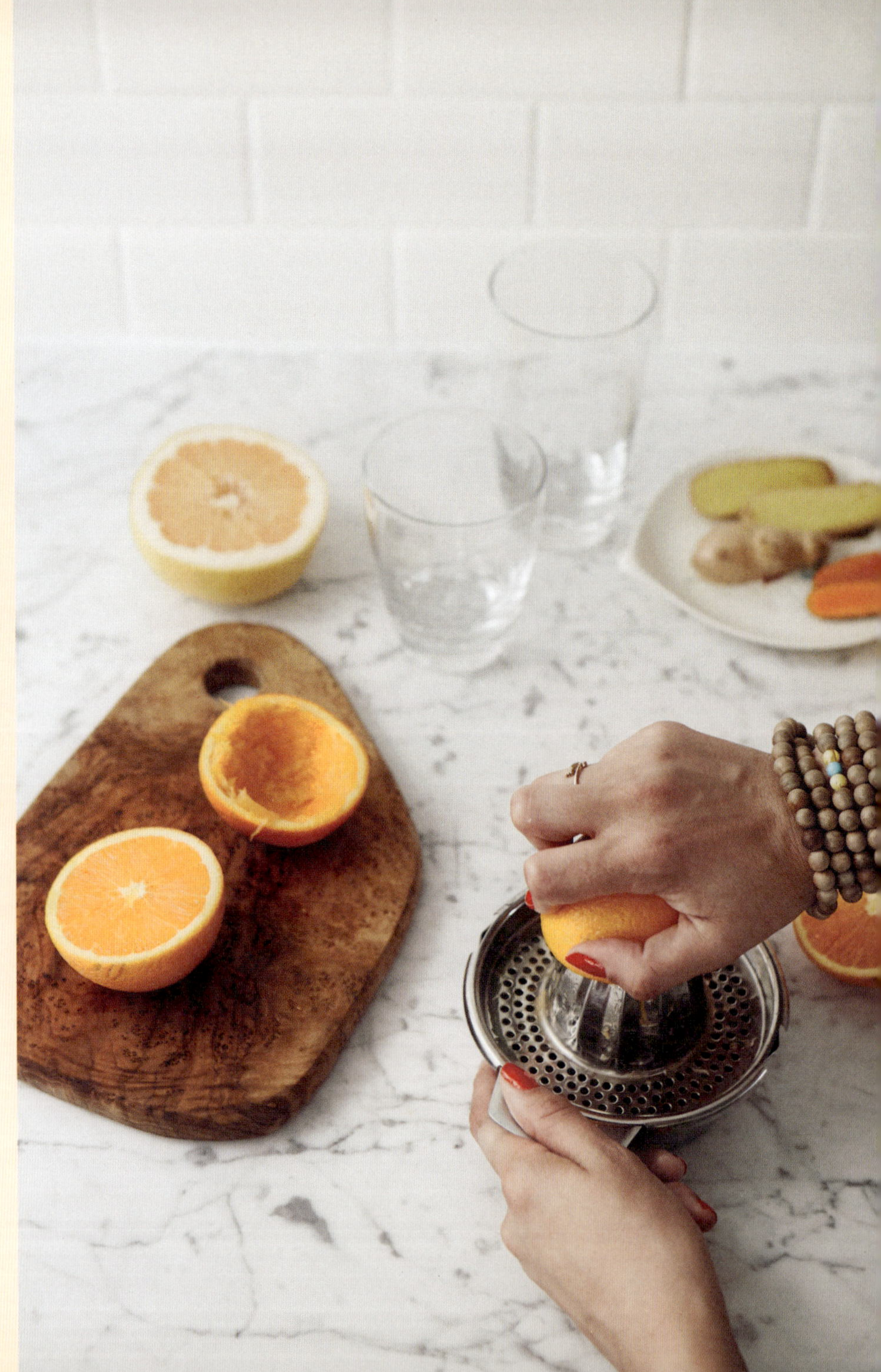

HOW TO USE THIS BOOK

Recipes

The recipes in this book have been designed to engage you in a mindful experience with what's on your plate. Each recipe has its own assigned affirmation (e.g., *My beauty radiates from within. I honor my basic needs. I choose to do things I love.*), which is purposefully paired with a specific meditation or mindfulness exercise. You may use them in any way you want, but I suggest choosing a recipe from this book that appeals to you, preparing the dish, and then reading the affirmation. Ponder it. Entertain the idea that perhaps being drawn to that specific recipe was indeed a way to bring you to that message. You can read the affirmation in the morning before you start cooking or in the evening after you've finished.

Though I don't endorse a specific diet, I do believe as a whole we can all benefit tremendously from incorporating more organic, plant-based meals into our diets. All of the recipes in this book are vegan. If your body is craving animal products, it's easy to substitute eggs and dairy back into all these recipes. You can also add additional protein to the salads, bowls, and mains if desired.

I encourage you to buy organic ingredients whenever possible. If they are not available or affordable for you, just be sure to thoroughly wash your fruit and veggies to rinse off any trace chemicals. Don't stress about it, just do your best! Overall, my mission is to get you eating more of the good stuff and having a better relationship with what's on your plate!

Meditation 101

I am a big advocate of a daily meditation and mindfulness practice. I and many of my clients have found it nothing short of life-changing. Start where you are comfortable, even if it's just for one minute a day, but don't be afraid to turn up your practice to correspond with your current needs. When you are starting out, it might be easiest to meditate right after waking up. Just sit up in bed and take those first few minutes of the day for yourself. When I first began, I was in a lot of emotional pain and found it helpful to meditate multiple times a day. Make your practice your own and take your time experimenting with what feels best for you. You'll find all different kinds of meditations paired with the recipes in this book, everything from your standard sit-down-with-a-mantra to walking, bath time, and nature meditations. This was intentional to give you a variety of entry points to find a practice that works for you and resonates with the goals that are most important to you right now. For example, if you want to improve your relationship with your body, then you might want to do a meditation where you express gratitude for all that your body does for you every single day. (And yes, that one's in here too!)

A Note on Gluten-Free Flour

All gluten-free flours have slightly different weight conversions. I use Bob's Red Mill Gluten Free 1-to-1 Baking Flour in my recipes.

WHAT DOES IT MEAN TO EAT WITH INTENTION?

Have you ever made cupcakes and accidentally screwed up the batter? Maybe you used an incorrect amount of flour or baking powder, and your cake turned out a bit wonky. Instead of throwing out the batter and starting all over, you made the most incredible frosting and slathered it on top. *Voilà!* Though you managed to disguise the problem, you didn't actually fix the cake.

Well, every time you try the latest diet craze—whether it's low-carb, paleo, keto, or whatever—you're hiding the cake. It's why you constantly feel frustrated when it comes to your body and the food you are putting in it. It's why dieting is always so hard and feels like a chore. Often, after you successfully lose a few pounds, you gain it back plus some. In this book, I will show you how to make peace with your body, heal your relationship with food, and eat with intention. I will help you fix the cake.

Eating with intention is the deceptively simple name for a process that involves shifting the relationship between food and your body. It means eating from a place of self-love and awareness. And I don't mean that fake, pretend self-love you see all over social media dressed up as bright pink quotes and selfies with flowers; I'm talking about that deep self-love that comes when you genuinely heal the relationship with your body and connect to your soul.

In this book, I will share my thoughts on the types of nourishment our bodies crave as well as delicious recipes to help us satisfy those cravings. However, learning the process of making peace with yourself, healing the unhealthy patterns you have around food, and listening to your body—so that it can tell you what it actually needs for nourishment, how much rest it needs, and how much to move and sweat—is far more valuable. *Your* body knows what it needs better than anyone else, including me. Our bodies are highly intelligent, and we need to respect and honor that wisdom. So how do you begin eating with intention?

After reflecting on my own experience around food and self-love, I realized there are four main pillars of the journey: making peace with your body, starting a conversation, becoming a food detective, and eating with intention. I use the term *pillars*, and not *steps*, because this isn't necessarily a linear process. You may find one pillar a more comfortable place to start than another. And even when you feel like you have mastered all four pillars, a bad habit could rear its ugly head again a few years down the road.

Think of these four pillars as your toolbox, and use them to bring yourself back to your truth. Learn them now to transform your relationship with your body, and keep them in a safe place in case any loose screws need a little tightening down the road.

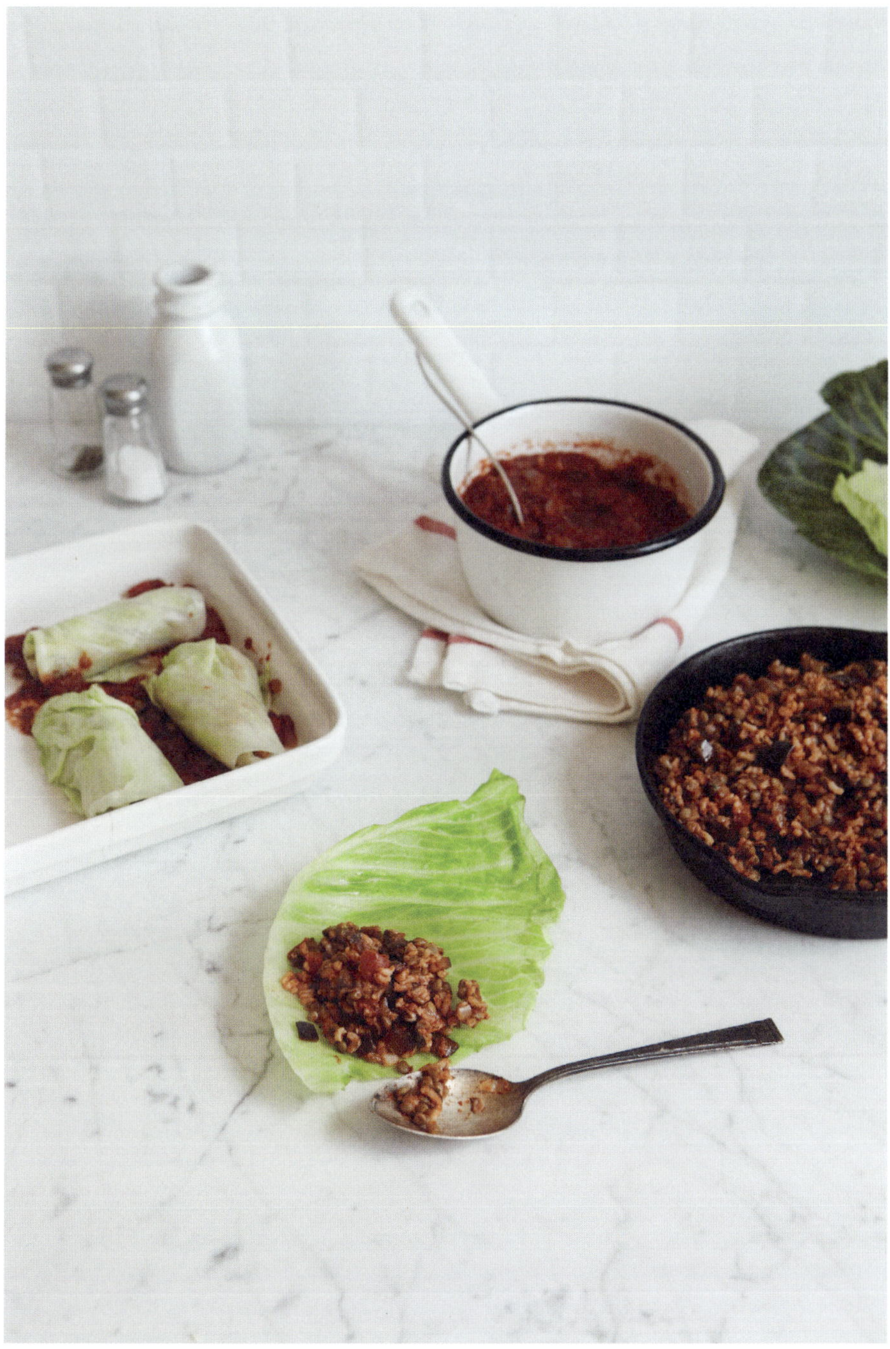

Pillar 1:
Making Peace with Your Body

Most of us are programmed to fight against our body. That's why all sorts of extreme dieting methods, hunger-reducing or metabolism-boosting pills, weight-loss injections, crazy exercise routines, and fat-removing surgeries are growing more popular in our culture. When we think of our body as an opponent, we have a conditional level of love for it: "I will love my body *after* this juice cleanse, because I will be less bloated and lose that excess weight." or "I will love my body *after* this 90-day cardio-and-ab challenge because I'll finally have a defined stomach."

Now, what if you shifted to thinking of your body like your partner's body? What if you loved your body the same way you love a life partner? I mean it's here for the long haul, right? Maybe your significant other's body isn't perfect, but I bet you would never make that a condition of your love for them. In fact, when we love from an unconditional place, we give people the freedom to become the best version of themselves on their own accord. Unconditional love has the power to transform—mind, body, and soul.

GRATITUDE

A major component of having a peaceful, loving relationship with your body is gratitude. Some people might be used to expressing gratitude for different aspects of their lives like friends, family, nature, or spirituality. But if you want to improve your relationship with your body, then you need to express gratitude for all that your body does for you every single day.

After experiencing pregnancy and the birth of my son, Hudson, I was brought to an even more deeply woven facet of gratitude for my body. Watching my body grow my beautiful baby boy each month of my pregnancy was simply wild. Experiencing my body bringing him into the world during my home birth was one of the most transcendental experiences of my life. Yet, even with all that magnificent, awe-inspiring magic, loving and listening to my new postpartum body has not been effortless. I've had to utilize the tools I teach in this book and consciously reconnect to my gratitude as I give my body the time and nourishment it needs to heal and find its new shape. (If you'd like to read more about this journey, grab the bonus chapter at *cassandrabodzak.com/themindfultable.*)

So please, don't chastise yourself if you can intellectually understand how grateful you are for your body but still struggle with negative thoughts about it during the day. There's nothing wrong with you. These practices are here to help you turn that intellectual understanding into a soul-deep knowing.

A body-gratitude meditation practice is a great way to become present and at home in your body. Take a few moments in the shower each morning to do an inventory of your body and say thank you for everything that you can. I'd say thank you for my beautiful legs that are strong and allow me to do yoga and walk all over the city with ease. Thank you for my stomach and intestines that allow me to process all the food I eat and give me loving nudges when I'm eating something that my body doesn't like. Thank you for my heart that beats every single day and centers me when I get too caught up in my thoughts. Thank you for my nose that allows me to smell the flowers and freshly baked cookies. You get the idea.

Be specific, be sincere, and choose things that feel authentic. So even if you don't like the size of your nose, perhaps you can express gratitude for the wonderful things it allowed you to smell today. If you want further inspiration, I've recorded an even more detailed guided meditation for deep body gratitude that you can listen to at *www.cassandrabodzak.com/themindfultable.* Spending a few minutes each day bowing to the miracles that naturally occur inside of you is essential to improving your relationship with your body.

END NEGATIVE SELF-TALK

The hardest part of making peace with your body is quieting that menacing negative self-talk. You know the kind I mean. The voice that tells you your thighs are too big. Or the one that calls you a pig after having pizza with your friends. While having a deep sense of love and appreciation for your body will lower the volume on that mean voice, you still need to actively stop yourself every single time you think or say something negative about your body. That voice is not the real you. In Michael Singer's *The Untethered Soul,* he compares this voice to a very rude roommate, and I love that analogy.

Stop Negative Thought Patterns

1. Pause. Take a few deep breaths.
2. Bring in your gratitude.
3. If you are struggling with Step 2, acknowledge that your nasty roommate is holding the mic right now. Feel free to talk back to it and put that voice in its place with a correction from your more self-loving perspective, or simply just tell it, "We are not going there right now."

LAUGHTER IS SPIRITUAL

If you feel tempted to judge yourself in a harsh or negative way, I urge you to remedy it with a nice big laugh at yourself. Laughing has become a deep spiritual practice for me. It instantly shifts the energy away from my inner critic and into a space of joy and deep love for myself.

This laughing technique is also a great weapon when it comes to negative self-talk. Let's say you are trying on that less-than-flattering bridesmaid's dress (surprise, surprise) that your friend picked out for you. As you look in the mirror, you suddenly hear that little voice start shouting, *If you lost five pounds, you would actually be able to zip this thing!* Before you continue down that path of self-abuse, hear it and try to see the situation from above—you are in the dressing room wearing a hideous dress and that annoying voice is telling you to lose weight! Take a moment to laugh at yourself and the absurdity of the situation! By laughing at those negative thought patterns, you disarm them, and they won't have the same power over you. So, laugh your beautiful face off, my dear!

I want to be clear here: Old thought patterns die hard, and this is a mindful muscle that you build over time. I also know that, sometimes, you break down in tears in the dressing room because that dress doesn't fit, and it just feels terrible. Trust me, I've been there. In those times, treat yourself as you would a best friend and care for yourself lovingly.

You may not always be able to silence your negative self-talk, but you can nip it in the bud before it bleeds into more destructive behaviors.

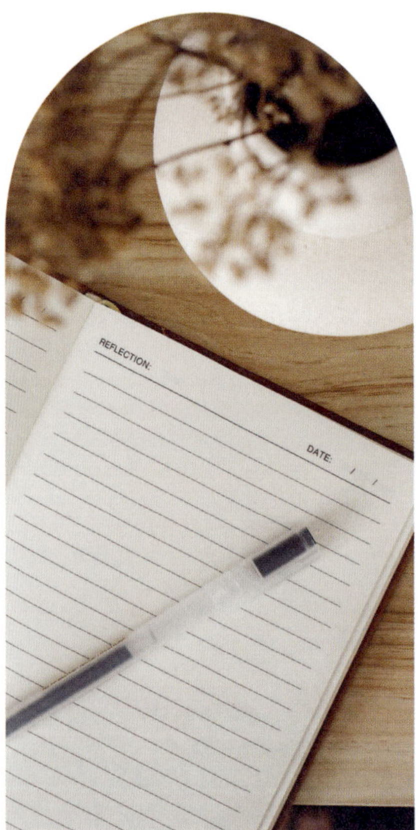

Pillar 2: Becoming a Food Detective

This next pillar involves becoming more aware of how the things we put into our body affect how it feels as we go about our daily lives. I call this process, "becoming a food detective." In my healing journey, becoming a food detective was the thing that saved me after many months of excruciating mystery pain—but this process is truly revelatory regardless of how you are feeling when you start. You'll be amazed at what you can uncover.

START A FOOD-MOOD JOURNAL

The first step involves bringing more awareness to *what* you are eating and *why* you are eating it. Start by keeping a food-mood journal. Many diets recommend regularly logging what you eat, but the food-mood journal is not about restriction or counting calories. Spending a few days becoming more aware of your food habits can be a big wake-up call. I have seen people realize almost immediately that they get a "dairy stomachache" after eating their yogurt or feel lethargic after their daily bacon-egg-and-cheese sandwich. Others reach for coffee and a donut in the mid-afternoon to wake up, but the sugar-caffeine jolt makes them feel worse. When you journal, you reveal these patterns.

The most important part of this pillar is that it is a *judgment-free* zone. I'm serious about this! Gathering this information is *not* meant to give more ammunition to that negative voice in your head. This is just data collection, so I beg you to look with compassion. We *all* have weird behaviors around food: places we go to on autopilot, or certain repeat indulgences. You are human, I am human, and I don't know if I could even trust a person who has never been tempted by leftover cookie dough in the fridge or scarfed down a heaping plate of fries!

Now we're ready to get down and dirty with the detective work here. Your food-mood journal can be any journal. You can jot down notes on your smartphone, download an app, or use a notebook that you can carry with you throughout the day.

THE TWO-WEEK FOOD-MOOD CHALLENGE

The real trick to this exercise is to *not* be on your best behavior around food for those two weeks. Don't behave like a starving college student at an all-you-can-eat buffet, but rather allow your regular habits to come through. You don't want to shift into hyper-clean eating for two weeks while you keep your log and then go right back to how you *actually* eat afterward.

Log Challenge!

For the next two weeks, after you complete your food-mood detective work, check in with your body before and after every meal. Before you decide what to put in your body, simply ask what it wants. We're often on autopilot around our food choices, even healthy ones. We get into a routine around what we eat for breakfast or lunch, and we don't check in with ourselves. One of our body's deepest needs is variety. It craves different foods because it needs all kinds of vitamins, minerals, and nutrients. When we become robots around our food choices, we deprive our body of this core desire. Remember, we are doing reps and building our intention muscles here, so really go for it: Ask your body for guidance. Push yourself to try this new way of operating. Ask about everything. If you are feeling tired or unfocused, ask about that too.

- Log *all* of your meals, snacks, and beverages! Yes, even that handful of M&M's at 3:30 p.m. during the staff meeting and the half of a gin and tonic you had during happy hour—everything! Don't cheat yourself here. The more honest you are, the clearer the picture will be of your regular diet. Also be sure to include things that you add to your food, like coconut milk in your coffee or sriracha on your avocado toast.
- Log how you feel before you eat the meal as well as how you feel 30 minutes to an hour post meal. For example, if you're feeling stressed when you head out to lunch, log it! And if you decide to eat a grilled cheese sandwich with tomato soup and then an hour later you are falling asleep at your desk, note it! No judgment here. We are just collecting valuable clues for your mind-body-food case.
- Log your focus and energy level throughout the day. You don't need to be super detailed, just note the big arcs, every four hours or so. This helps you see when in the day you are energized and when you are tired.

If you ever notice a sudden dip in energy or mood, bloating, or any other uncomfortable symptom, know that you can put your food-mood journal back into play. Some people will bring it when they go away on a trip because it helps them see what foods are working for them as they introduce different meals, remove certain ingredients, and incorporate different activities into their life.

THE RESULTS ARE IN!

After your initial two weeks, sit down with your log and a few colored highlighters. Highlight all the times you felt extremely exhausted with one color, then go back and see if there are any similarities in the foods you ate on those days. Perhaps you notice that every time you eat a sandwich for lunch, you can barely keep your eyes open after 2 p.m., but on the days you eat a salad, it's not nearly as intense. Take a different color highlighter and note all the instances you felt sick or had a stomachache. Look for patterns. Did you have a common food like dairy or gluten before all your stomach issues? Don't overwhelm yourself by trying to find every single thing in your diet or lifestyle habits that may be causing you some discomfort. Trust me, there will be plenty of time for you to keep refining!

When I go over food-mood logs with clients, I laser in on the top three issues based on the patterns I see in behavior, mood, and ingredients. Pay attention to your body. Any time you experience physical pain or a total lack of energy or focus, you can probably transform your experience by making some simple swaps in your diet or routine. Take action on one to two patterns at a time. For example, you might decide to remove dairy from your diet and see if that eliminates any stomachaches you were experiencing. That one adjustment is plenty to start. If I noticed that I regularly feel bloated and exhausted after I eat, then I could also potentially try to be more conscious about slowing down and chewing my food completely during meals. Whatever you deduce, commit to the elimination or change for the next three weeks and notice what happens. Did the stomachaches vanish as soon as the dairy did? How were your energy levels affected once you started eating slower?

Most importantly, honor the observations in your diet and get into the habit of communicating with your body. Which brings me to the third pillar—starting a conversation.

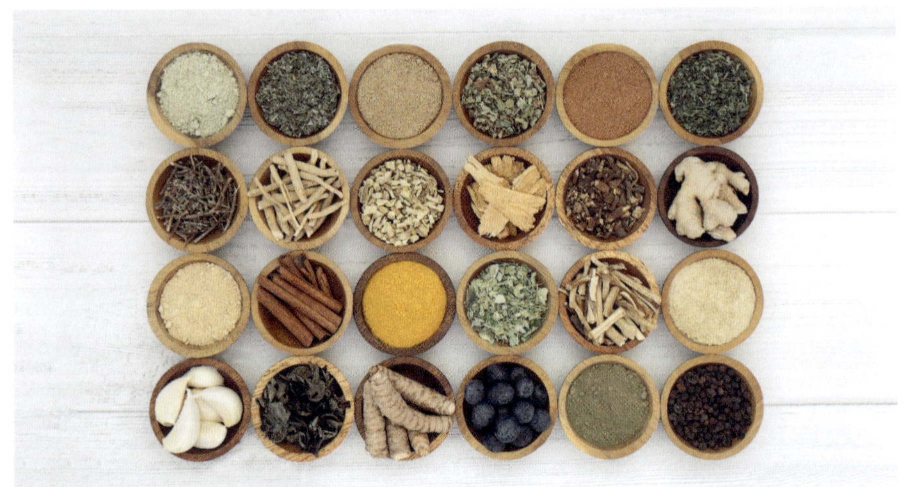

Pillar 3:
Starting a Conversation

When was the last time you really sat down, tuned in, and had a heart-to-heart with your body? It might sound odd to "meet and go over everything," but talking to your body can be a transformative experience. Our bodies are brilliant and know exactly what they need to run at their best.

Personally, I never wanted to put tomatoes or peppers into anything I cooked. When I was tested for food allergies, I discovered that tomatoes and peppers were inflammatory for my body. I listen to my body now, and I trust what it's trying to tell me.

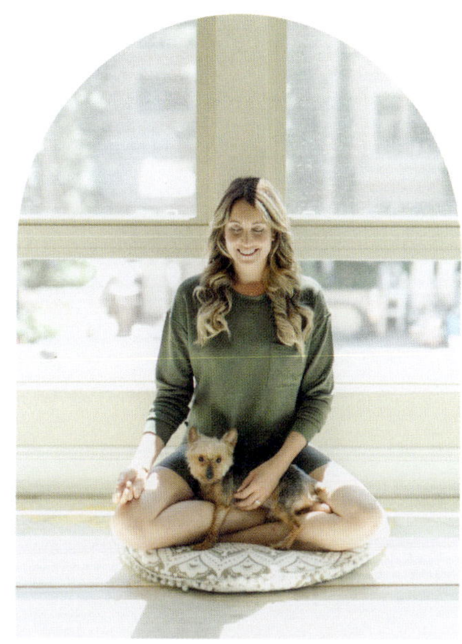

THE FIRST STEPS

Let's start at the beginning. Try the meditation below to open up the channels of communication with your body:

Close your eyes, place your hands on your heart, and take a few long, deep breaths. Release any tension, stress, or strain and allow any thoughts to pass by like clouds. Bring yourself back to your breath, back to your body. Now ask your body silently, how have I been treating you? What do you need to feel your best? How can I take better care of you? Allow silence after each question to give yourself the space to hear the answers. Keep a notebook nearby if you feel the need to write anything down. Honor whatever it is you hear.

This might feel awkward at first, and that's perfectly fine. We are building a lifelong partnership here. The most important thing is to ask your body questions and allow yourself to hear the answers. As you get better at listening to your body, this "check-in" can become more casual, just a deep breath in and an honest question. Keep it simple so you can do it anywhere, whether you're out at a restaurant or shopping in the supermarket. The point is to start an ongoing dialogue with your body so that you know what it needs and how best to take care of it.

Though it is not always obvious, your body is constantly feeding you data. Pay attention to your body language the next time you are with someone—if your shoulders drop, your heart center opens, and your general energy feels relaxed, your body is giving you a spiritual thumbs up. If you feel your shoulders curl inward, and your body tense up, it's giving you a "no." You can use this test for all sorts of decisions. Place your hands on your heart and visualize yourself in a situation; feel how your body responds. In the framework of food, picture yourself eating a particular dish and feel how that dining experience sits with your body.

FORGET THE LABELS AND JUST LISTEN

I have never felt very connected to the labels *vegan* or *gluten-free*. In fact, I encourage my clients to forget labels and just listen. However, I do want to take a moment to address two recent diet crazes: keto and high protein.

I believe deeply in "bio-individuality." Each body is unique. We have different ancestry, genetic expressions, trauma, microbiomes, lifestyles, stress levels, and underlying conditions that impact how our bodies run, which foods fuel us best, how much rest we need, and more. Your phase of life is also a factor—for example, if you're menstruating, pre, or post-menopausal, different foods, exercises, and supplements are going to be supportive for you. We can make a few broad statements. For example, eating a lot of refined sugar is not great for your health. But we have to be careful when following a strict diet plan that's not tailored to our body's needs.

So, how do we navigate food trends? We honor our curiosity and interest, we go into our food detective mode, and we allow ourselves to explore. Tuning into your body and observing how different foods make you feel will arm you with the confidence to take in whatever dietary advice might be floating around and pick out what works for you. I'm happy to share my own observations to help you get started:

The keto diet is based on eating a significant amount of fat and a good amount of protein. I've had some clients thrive on keto and others for whom it wasn't a good fit. Once again, I encourage you to take the driver's seat. I do love that keto gets people away from counting calories and focuses instead on the macronutrients in the food they are eating. This is fabulous for us all. It also has you eliminating a lot of junk from your diet. Bye-bye refined sugars and flours! However, I do not love how it also leads people to sometimes avoid antioxidant-packed fruits and stop filling up their bowls with nutrient-dense root veggies and grounding starches because of the low carb count needed to sustain ketosis. When eliminating nutrient-void snack foods, most people will feel better right off the bat. Unfortunately, because keto has become so popular, there are now a multitude of highly processed, not-so-healthy "sugar-free" keto products on the shelf.

Similarly, the high-protein trend is great at getting people back to eating real, whole foods and stepping away from overly processed substances. There's a lot of flexibility for how you get that protein, so you can decide what feels best for you. Protein is in broccoli and spinach, chickpeas, lentils, quinoa, tofu, edamame, beans, and animal products. There is a whole spectrum to choose from! However, the amount of protein that each person needs varies widely based on an individual's health and lifestyle. If you are always hungry or reaching for a snack between meals, focusing on protein can bring you more peace by satiating your appetite. Just don't forget to include lots of nutrient-packed organic fruits and veggies on your menu! Also, pay attention to how a high-protein meal makes you feel at different parts of the day—for some people a big protein-packed breakfast feels amazing; others might feel sluggish because their body wants a lighter start.

Ultimately, I want you to make your own rules and allow your body to ask for what it needs on a moment-to-moment basis. If you feel super empowered and energized by a particular diet, whether it's paleo, vegan, keto, or Mediterranean, then go for it. But as someone who came from a place of restriction, I believe labels may set pre-established guidelines that stop you from listening and communicating with your body. I derive great freedom from knowing that I can eat anything I want, that nothing is off limits, and that I can come to my plate each day with deep love and acceptance. That label-free mentality keeps me effortlessly plant-based without feeling like I'm missing out on something.

I work with people all over the world with all kinds of eating preferences, and I would never dream of pushing a specific diet on any of them. My role is to stimulate a conversation so grounded in deep love and respect that they receive the guidance they need to fuel their bodies for optimal performance each and every day. I have complete and utter confidence in each one of your bodies to lead you along the path to radiant health and the foods that will help you get there.

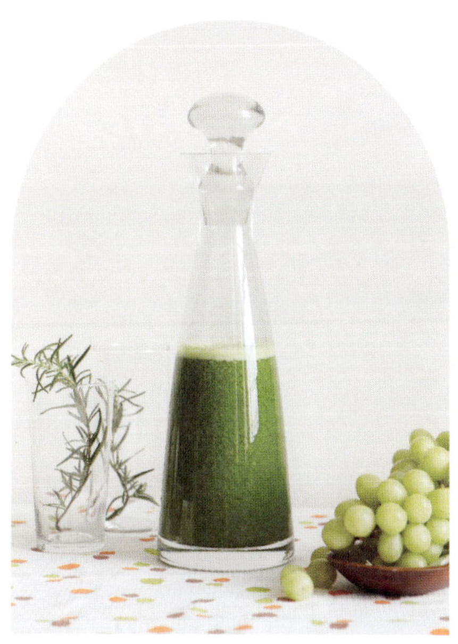

THE CRAVE CURE

If you are anything like I once was, you believe your cravings are the archenemy in the battle for a healthy, vibrant body. I used to abhor my cravings, but being in a loving, open relationship with my body meant that I needed to listen to and interpret my cravings. For example, when I had a french fry craving that wouldn't go away, I honored it, and I ended up ordering them every single night for a week. When I still found myself yearning for fries after the week was up, I realized I needed to understand the root of this powerful craving. So, I closed my eyes, put my hands on my heart, and asked my body what it *really* wanted.

As I listened, it all made sense. My body wanted something grounding. It was craving root vegetables—like potatoes—to feel balanced and centered. I had automatically interpreted this request as fries because I wasn't in the habit of eating root vegetables like carrots, beets, or potatoes. After checking in with my body, I made myself hearty dinners that included roasted carrots or thinly sliced roasted potatoes and started feeling better immediately, and all those french fry cravings vanished.

Communicating with our bodies isn't always simple and direct. Sometimes we have to do some decoding, particularly when it comes to our cravings, because our minds will go to the most readily available example. If you take the time to break down your cravings, you will learn about your body's needs. A good way to do this is by asking yourself why consuming a particular food would make you feel good? This usually gets down to the source of the craving. And instead of leaping to the easiest or fastest solution, think about a few alternatives to those cravings that might help fulfill that underlying need.

Pillar 4:
Falling in Love with Food

If you have ever been on a diet, a meal plan, a juice cleanse, or anything similar, then the idea of falling in love with your food probably feels a little dangerous. It certainly terrified me. I have always loved food, but I felt that enjoying food was some kind of evil urge that I needed to control at all times. I could not unleash it, or it might completely destroy me. I never bothered to try new things or get creative in the kitchen because food was the enemy, and our relationship was strictly business.

After years of creative practice, however, I am delighted to tell you that there is a better way. You can fall in love with food that is both delicious *and* nourishes your body. When you practice tremendous gratitude and love for your body, when you start a conscious conversation to navigate its needs and decode its cravings, and when you treat your body like the precious gift it is, something magical happens. You start to fall in love with the act of fueling it.

SACRED COOKING

Making your kitchen a sacred space is a key part of eating with intention. Your kitchen is where it all begins: It's where you can create food that can heal, nourish, and energize. When you walk into your kitchen, you should be filled with a sense of joy. For me, this means clean counters, cute measuring cups, and a bright white kitchen flooded with daylight. For years, I couldn't swing the big white kitchen with lots of windows, but I made my tiny kitchen feel more desirable by keeping it clean and tidy, having fresh flowers on the windowsill, and really appreciating the light. Work with what you have! Something as simple as buying pretty oven mitts and dish towels can extend some of your personality to your kitchen. If your kitchen feels overstocked, cluttered, or off-balance, try a full cabinet and fridge clean-out. After you finish, you will feel lighter in every sense.

By infusing the whole preparation process with love, you will inevitably infuse your food with love. When I cook, I give my full, undivided attention to the process. I play mantras or a fun, upbeat playlist, depending on my mood that day. I get out all the ingredients I want to play with. I set up my brightly colored mixing bowls, my decorative whale-motif measuring cups, and my gold anchor spoons to bring fun and energy to the process. And then I just dive in and stay present with each step. I promise that if you do this, meal preparation becomes its own meditation. When you're chopping vegetables, stay present for the chopping, and give yourself over to this process. When sautéing, stay there with the spatula in your pan. If other thoughts or worries pop up, just redirect your focus back to the pan, back to the cooking. This way of preparing food will bring a whole new level of deliciousness to your meals and your mind.

Additionally, if you put love and care into making your food look as beautiful and delicious as it tastes, you will feel more nourished and satisfied. Take smoothie bowls, for example. Would you rather drink a greenish-brown liquid before your morning workout or eat a gorgeous bowl with granola, superfood sprinkles, berries, bananas—all working harmoniously in an eye-catching design? I love this dressed-up version of the smoothie! The presentation of your food matters, even if you're making a quick breakfast for one. When you put effort into plating your food, you foster reverence and respect for the food you ingest.

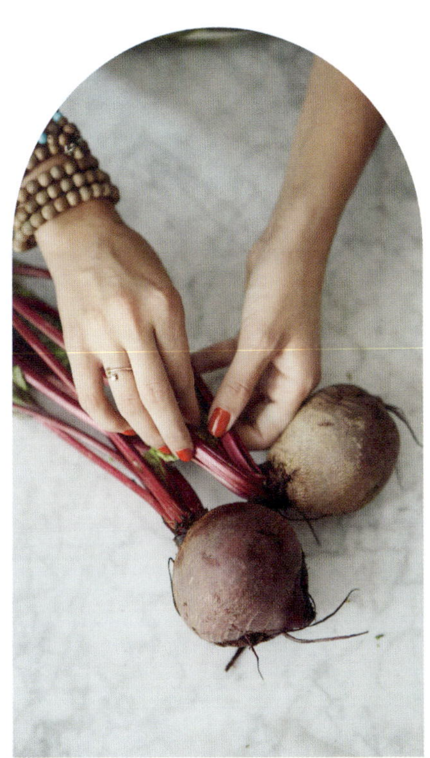

EAT MINDFULLY

This leads me right into mindful, intentional eating. Once you've developed a healthy sense of gratitude and acceptance for your body, practiced eating from a place of self-love, and begun an ongoing dialogue with your body—mindful eating just happens! If you are already connected and in tune with the process, mindful eating becomes a default setting. Magic, right?

Want to delve deeper? Set specific intentions for your food at every meal and engage in conscious chewing practices to make your eating even more mindful. Sit down, close the laptop, put the phone away, and focus on your food. When you are eating, eat without distractions. Eat with purpose. Take the time to engage with your food and savor each bite. Your stomach doesn't have teeth, so chewing your food well will improve digestion and keep you present with the delicious meal in front of you. If you are naturally a quick eater, break the cycle by putting your fork down after each bite; finish chewing before you pick it up again. Establishing the space and time to enjoy your food will slow you down and allow you to value the experience.

Ask yourself before each meal whether you are eating from a place of self-love or self-sabotage. Think about a time when you were particularly upset or stressed out, and even though you were eating the same normal foods you always eat, they were going right through you or giving you a stomachache. When we are in certain emotional and energetic states, our bodies have a much harder time digesting food. The energy with which you eat can affect the way your body processes that food.

So, what should you do when you're eating something from a place of self-sabotage and not self-love? The first step is to have a conversation with yourself as to why you are eating what's on your plate. Then, you can proceed in one of two ways:

You might acknowledge that you are eating the food in front of you in a self-sabotaging manner because you don't love your body right now and you want it to be different. Take a moment to search for that place of gratitude for your body. Once you achieve that, continue with your food from a place of self-awareness. This small acknowledgment can be enough to cause a shift in your intention and energy around the food.

The second way—and what I recommend doing when you're starting out—is to ask yourself if the food in front of you is what you really want. Ask yourself, "If I fully loved and accepted my body, what would I have in this moment?" Give yourself permission to have it. Sometimes you will hear your body telling you that it wants a smoothie, other times you will hear that it wants a more substantial breakfast. I love asking that question because even if it's just a hypothetical, you are pausing in the moment and tuning in to what it would feel like to genuinely love and accept your body. Keep practicing and building that self-love!

When you eat from a place of self-love, you bring more awareness around your specific intention for that meal: nourishment, healing, or energy.

ALIGN YOUR PLATE WITH THE SEASONS

Our bodies have different rhythms, not just in different phases of our lives, but in different literal seasons. This is why the recipes in this book are organized into thematic sections for fall, winter, spring, and summer. Of course, you can enjoy any of these recipes at any point of the year, but there is something beautiful (and delicious!) about aligning our plates with the Earth's seasons.

After all, we naturally crave a warm bowl of soup in the winter to keep us cozy from the inside out. We reach for that refreshing watermelon slice on a hot afternoon at the beach. Your body's wisdom is attuned to these patterns, all you need to do is listen to it.

Choosing seasonal foods not only helps your body sync up with the climate around you, but it also means that you will be eating fruits and vegetables at the peak of both their flavor and nutrient value. I highly recommend taking yourself on a date to your local farmer's market once a month (or more!) to experience the changing crops of fruits and produce in real time. You can observe how you are naturally drawn to different items on different days and allow your body to speak to you in this way as well.

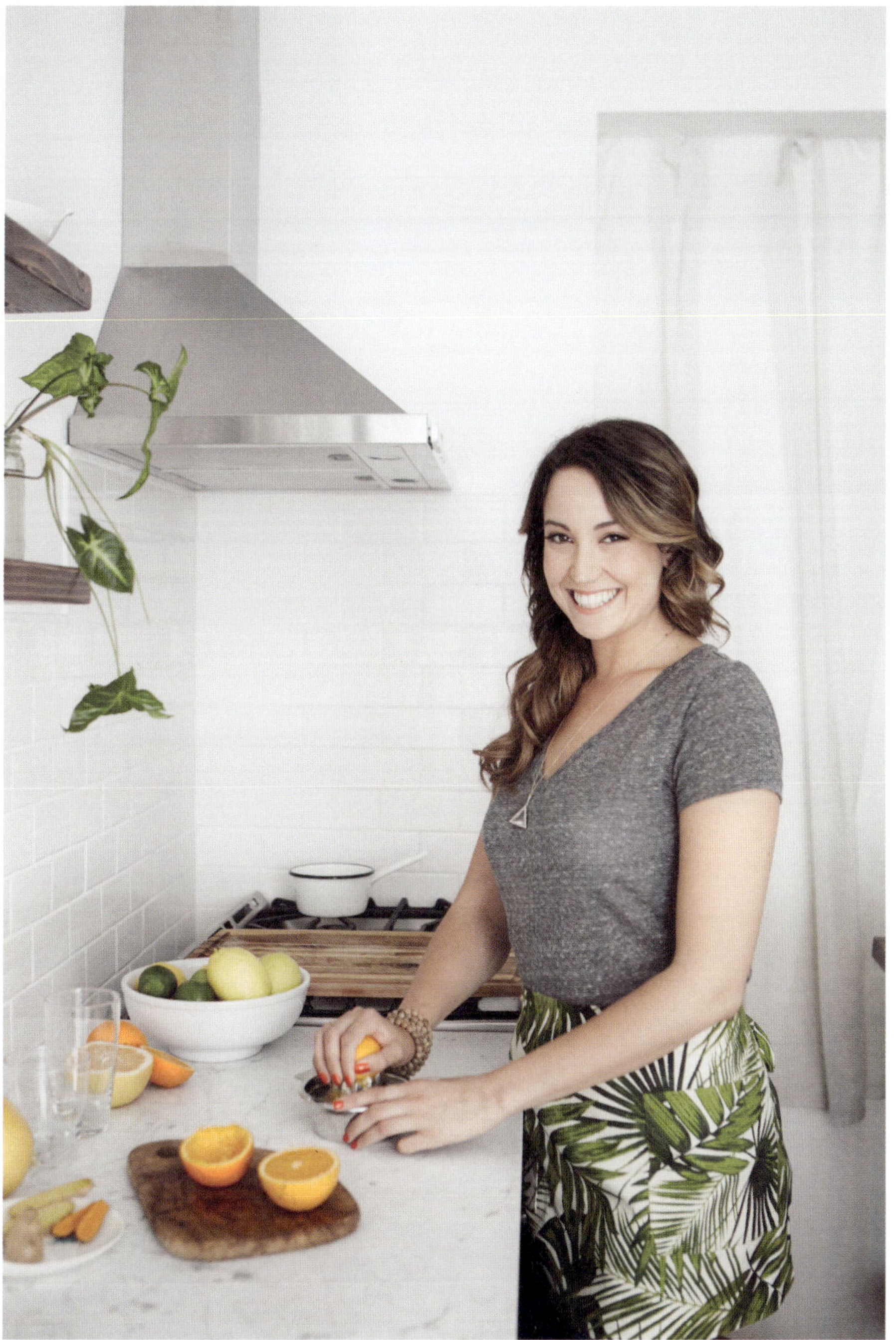

TRIGGERS AND TROUBLESHOOTING

If you find that you're sometimes uncomfortable sticking to your new mindful eating habits, that makes perfect sense. Your old habits kept you safe, but they also kept you from experiencing self-growth. There is going to be a learning curve. I urge you to enjoy it! Laugh through it. Be kind to yourself during this transition. You are retraining your mind and your body.

Your old patterns and habits around food and your body will not vanish overnight. Luckily, with persistent effort and consciousness around your behaviors, you will rewrite those old patterns with new ones. Here, I share some tools for maintaining this new way of life.

When Should I Stop Eating a Food Altogether?

At times, abstinence is required when it comes to eating habits. I have no trouble limiting gluten in my life: Having bread as an infrequent indulgence makes it easier for me to avoid it the rest of the time. Sugar, on the other hand, is my guilty pleasure. When I eat a little bit, I can barely stop myself from eating it five more times that day. If I bake cookies that aren't sugar-free, I will eat them all. They don't stand a chance.

The trick is to know what foods trigger you. What foods stir up addictive behaviors in you, or lead you further down a destructive rabbit hole? These foods are *not* your friends. Can you think of anything you're currently eating that has this kind of effect on you? If you think you know your "trigger" foods, jot them down in your food-mood journal. Pay some extra attention to them this week and observe your patterns around these foods, so you can decide whether to abstain from them altogether.

It's important to be brutally honest with yourself during this process. Do some journaling and let it all out. You are not weird. You are not weak. You are human—and you are incredibly brave and courageous for having the fortitude to look at yourself and your habits. You are ready to rewrite that programming!

Cold Turkey

Once you've identified a problem food, some people find it easiest to give it all up at once. But you can also take a gradual approach if that works best for you. Eliminating in stages may also lessen the pain of the detox.

If your trigger food is sugar, start off by eliminating added sugar (like the kind you might put in your coffee) and sweet treats like cupcakes and cookies. Once you begin to feel comfortable, start to read the labels of your groceries and avoid anything that contains sneaky "dried cane syrup" or "high fructose corn syrup." I've found it in almond milk, granola, salad dressings, and other unassuming foods, but it can be overwhelming to tackle all that when you first begin.

The one thing I do not recommend during this process is giving yourself a "cheat day" with your trigger food, because it will make it exponentially harder for you to abstain the remaining six days of the week and may lead you to binge on that one day. You wouldn't tell an alcoholic that it was okay to drink on Sundays, or that having one glass of wine with dinner doesn't count. Be honest with yourself, go inside, and determine if any foods or beverages (like coffee!) make you feel this way.

Situation Triggers

What situations lead you to abnormally excessive food consumption? Where do you feel you lose control or get caught up in a habitual pattern and feel powerless to resist?

Alcohol was a major trigger for me, and I see it with many friends and clients too. It's easy to see why: Alcohol impairs our judgment, which means we are not making our most intuitive choices when we are tipsy. When you're beginning to incorporate new patterns of eating, abstain from triggers such as alcohol to make it easier to commit to the change. With time and awareness, I was able to have an occasional glass of wine without getting derailed. Know yourself and make the choice that's going to set you up for success!

Holidays, barbecues, and buffets can be triggers because of the copious options and your sense of obligation to try a bit of everything. As a result, you end up eating way more than you needed and feel guilty and uncomfortable. When faced with a buffet, give yourself two plates. Fill your first plate up with all the salad you want, and let the second plate be your "main course." This is a little visual trick to help your brain register that you have eaten an entire meal. Trying a little of this and a little of that with ten tiny plates doesn't give us the visual cue to stop eating or help us feel full.

Emotional Eating During Stressful Times

The final trigger I want to mention is stress. Many people tend to eat emotionally during stressful situations. Maybe you have a habit of stopping by the bakery on your way home from work and "treating" yourself to a red velvet cupcake when you've had a stressful day. These eating patterns have become cultural norms, so we've become oblivious to the fact that we have ritualized our emotional eating. We try to eat away our feelings and numb the pain we are going through instead of dealing with the feelings that are coming up for us.

What would happen if you treated yourself with love during those rough emotional times? If you asked yourself what you really needed? Maybe it's a walk outside to unwind from the day, to listen to a guided meditation to recalibrate, or to call a friend to catch up. I guarantee that it is not really a pint of ice cream.

One great tool for averting stress-induced eating habits is mindful meal planning. Meal planning takes you off of autopilot and relieves pressure to make food decisions in the moment, when you might be distracted or distressed from the day's trials. If you find the constant debate about where to eat or what to make for your next meal exhausting, plan it out the night before! Save your precious time and brain space and relax about the food.

01

Spring

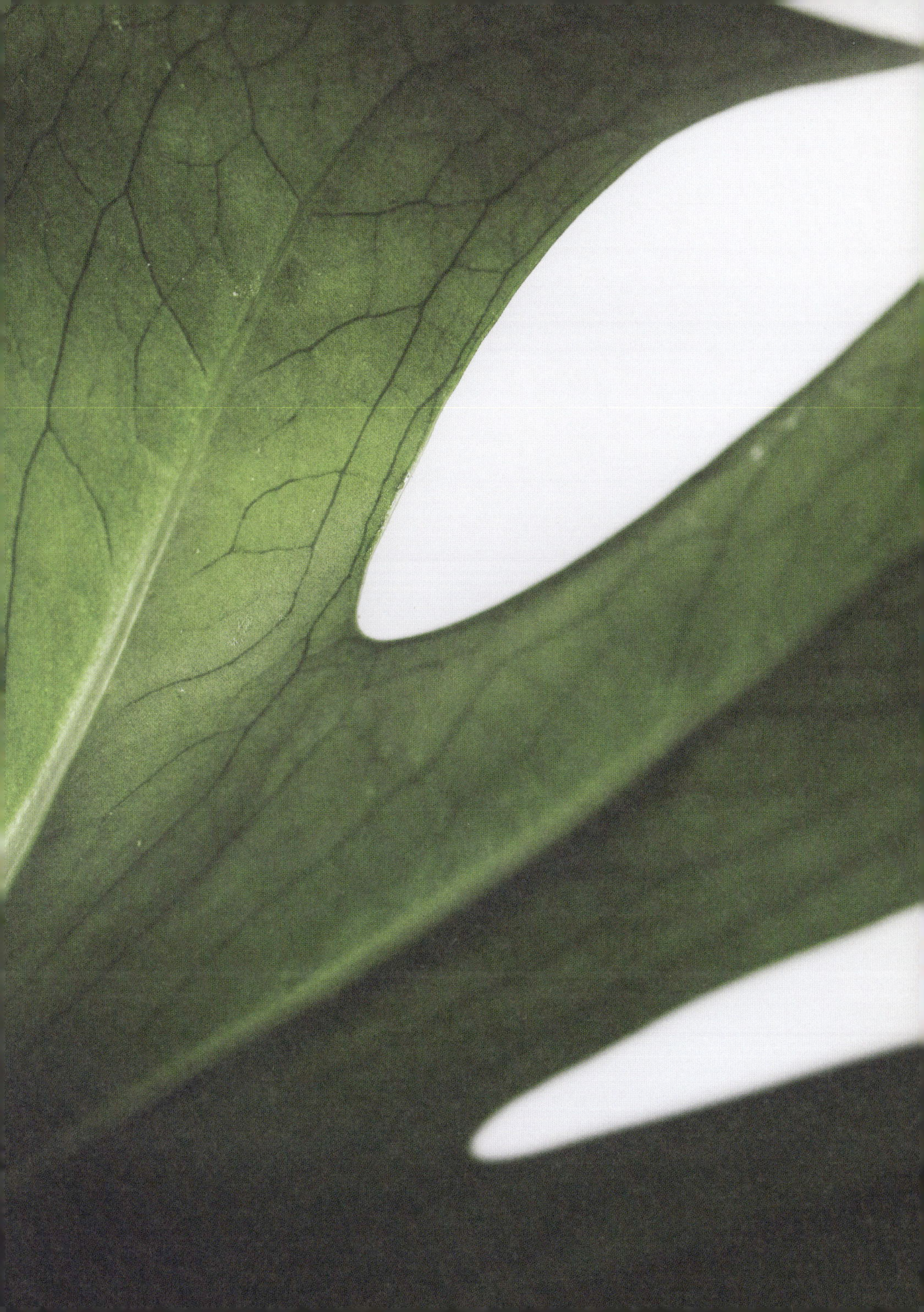

Berry Green Smoothie

How we view our life is a matter of perspective, and it's often far easier for us to focus on the negative and throw the scales off balance. This is why a daily mindfulness practice like alternate nostril breathing is helpful in bringing our awareness back into balance so we can see the full picture. This smoothie is a great example of that delicate balance: It has good-for-you greens; tart, antioxidant-packed berries; and a sweet creaminess from the banana and almond butter.

YIELD: 1 serving

1 banana
1 cup (240 ml) unsweetened almond milk
½ cup (93 g) frozen mixed berries
½ cup (34 g) chopped kale or spinach
1 tablespoon (16 g) of your favorite nut butter
1 heaping teaspoon reishi mushroom powder (optional)

Combine all the ingredients in a blender and purée until thoroughly blended.

Pour into a large glass and serve immediately.

Kundalini Meditation for Perspective and Emotional Balance (alternate nostril breathing)

Sit comfortably with your eyes closed, focusing on your third-eye point (the space between your eyebrows). Use your right thumb and right pinkie (or thumb and index finger) to close off alternate nostrils. Close off the right nostril with your thumb. Inhale deeply through the left nostril. When the breath is full, close off the left nostril with your pinkie and exhale smoothly through the right nostril. The breath should be complete, continuous, and smooth. Continue for 3 minutes, gradually building up to 31 minutes. Close with a deep inhale, then an exhale, holding the breath out for a moment. Relax.

"

I have power over my perspective.

Focus Potion

This potion is a bit of a secret weapon of mine for days when shiny objects and social media are getting the better of me. The sweet combination of grapes with the alkalizing punch of kale and celery perks you up, while rosemary focuses all that magical energy! It combines beautifully with a divine purpose meditation, which allows us to tune out the noise and connect with what we're really here to do.

YIELD: 1 serving

3 celery stalks
2 cups (134 g) baby kale
1 cup (150 g) grapes
3 drops rosemary essential oil (food grade)
2 sprigs fresh rosemary, to garnish

Put celery, kale, and grapes into a juicer and juice into a large glass.

Stir in the rosemary oil, garnish with sprigs of rosemary, and serve immediately.

Divine Purpose Visualization

Sit comfortably with your eyes closed and focused on your third-eye point. Take long, deep breaths in through your nose and out through your mouth. Feel your body come into a calm balance. Now, bring your purpose on this planet to the top of your mind. (If you are unclear of what your purpose is, use ***I am here to embody pure love***, because that is all of our divine purpose.) Allow it to be your mantra for a few moments, letting it roll around your head, down your spine, and through your breath flow. Now bring to mind what this would look like to you. How do you behave? How do people around you feel and act? What's your ripple effect in the world? Allow these images to flood your mind for the next 3 to 5 minutes before bringing yourself back to your original purpose statement. Take a deep breath in, hold it, and release it.

"

I am focused on my divine purpose.

Unicorn Fuel

Whenever I'm feeling stuck, it's a sure sign I'm not attuned to my own magic. And when I want to draw on my magic, I need to proper magical fuel! This smoothie may taste like a piña colada, but it is extra powerful (hence the name "unicorn"). The accompanying meditation will help you unlock your own "magic wand," your Jupiter finger, and allow you to lean into the magic that's always been available to you.

YIELD: 1 serving

¼ cup (23 g) unsweetened shredded coconut, plus extra to garnish
1 cup (240 ml) unsweetened almond milk
½ cup (83 g) pineapple chunks, plus extra to garnish
1 tablespoon (12 g) raw extra-virgin coconut oil
1 teaspoon cordyceps mushroom powder
1 teaspoon vitamin C powder
1 teaspoon moringa leaf powder

Preheat the oven to 350°F (180°C, or gas mark 4). Spread the shredded coconut evenly on a baking sheet and bake for 7–8 minutes, stirring occasionally, until light golden brown.

Combine all the ingredients in a blender and purée until thoroughly blended. Fill a large glass with ice, add the juice, and garnish with pineapple chunks and toasted coconut, if desired. Serve immediately.

Waving Your Wand Meditation

Start seated, arms at your side, with your index fingers (or Jupiter fingers) pointing up to the sky or ceiling and the rest of your fingers in a fist. Close your eyes and bring your inner focus towards your third eye. Breathe into this space, feeling your index fingers as if they are your very own magical wands, shooting a command straight from your heart into the heavens. Feel your dreams and desires moving from your heart center, out your fingers, and up into the heavens. Sit and breathe here for 10 minutes as you channel all the desires in your heart, feeling them already being fulfilled.

To close, bring your hands together in prayer position at your heart center and sit in gratitude for a few minutes.

"
I'm attuned to my magic.

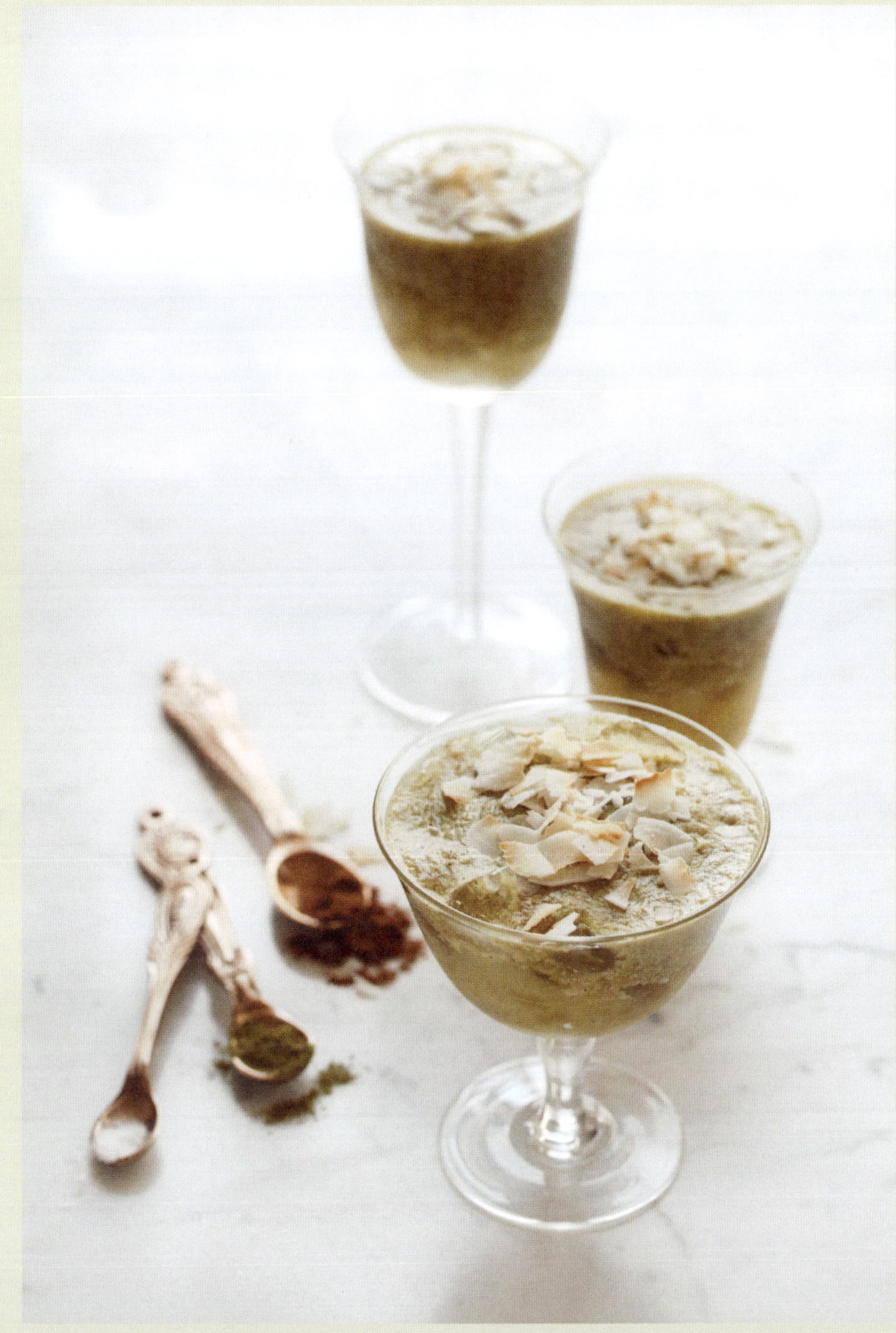

Avocado Toast Three Ways

We can't be well-oiled machines all of the time; our lives can get messy or chaotic, which is why it's so important to know ourselves and prepare accordingly. Avocado toast is one of those meals that has helped a lot of people find success with their diets. It's a super easy, filling, healthy, go-to breakfast or lunch. Plus, its limitless variations will have you feeling like a creative genius in the kitchen, giving you a boost in confidence just when you need it.

YIELD: 1 serving (per option)

OPTION 1

2 tablespoons (30 g) roasted garlic hummus
1 slice Ezekiel bread, toasted
1 avocado, halved, pitted, and sliced
½ cup (34 g) sautéed kale (see page 104)
½ cup (44 g) sautéed red onions
Pinch of salt
Pinch of freshly ground black pepper

OPTION 2

1 avocado, halved, pitted, and mashed
1 flatbread cracker (I love the seasoned ones from Wasa)
1 radish, thinly sliced
Spring peas, cooked
Drizzle of extra-virgin olive oil
Pinch of salt

OPTION 3

1 avocado, halved, pitted, and mashed
1 brown rice cake
1 fresh peach, sliced and sautéed in extra-virgin coconut oil

To make option 1, spread the hummus on the bread. Top with the sliced avocado, sautéed kale, and red onions, and season with a pinch of salt and pepper. Serve.

To make option 2, spread the mashed avocado on the flatbread. Arrange the sliced radish on top and scatter over the peas. Drizzle over the olive oil and season with salt. Serve.

To make option 3, spread the mashed avocado on the rice cake, then top with the peach slices. Serve.

Inner Superstar Visualization

Sit comfortably with your spine straight and your eyes closed. Imagine yourself going through the day ahead as your best self: You are sailing through the same meetings, tasks, errands, and interactions with ease, grace, confidence, and bliss. Go through your day and all the activities involved thoroughly and notice the energy that this "super star you" brings to each situation. When you've gone through your whole day, take a deep breath in. Hold it, allowing all of that magnificent energy to circulate within your body, then exhale.

"

I am rigged for success.

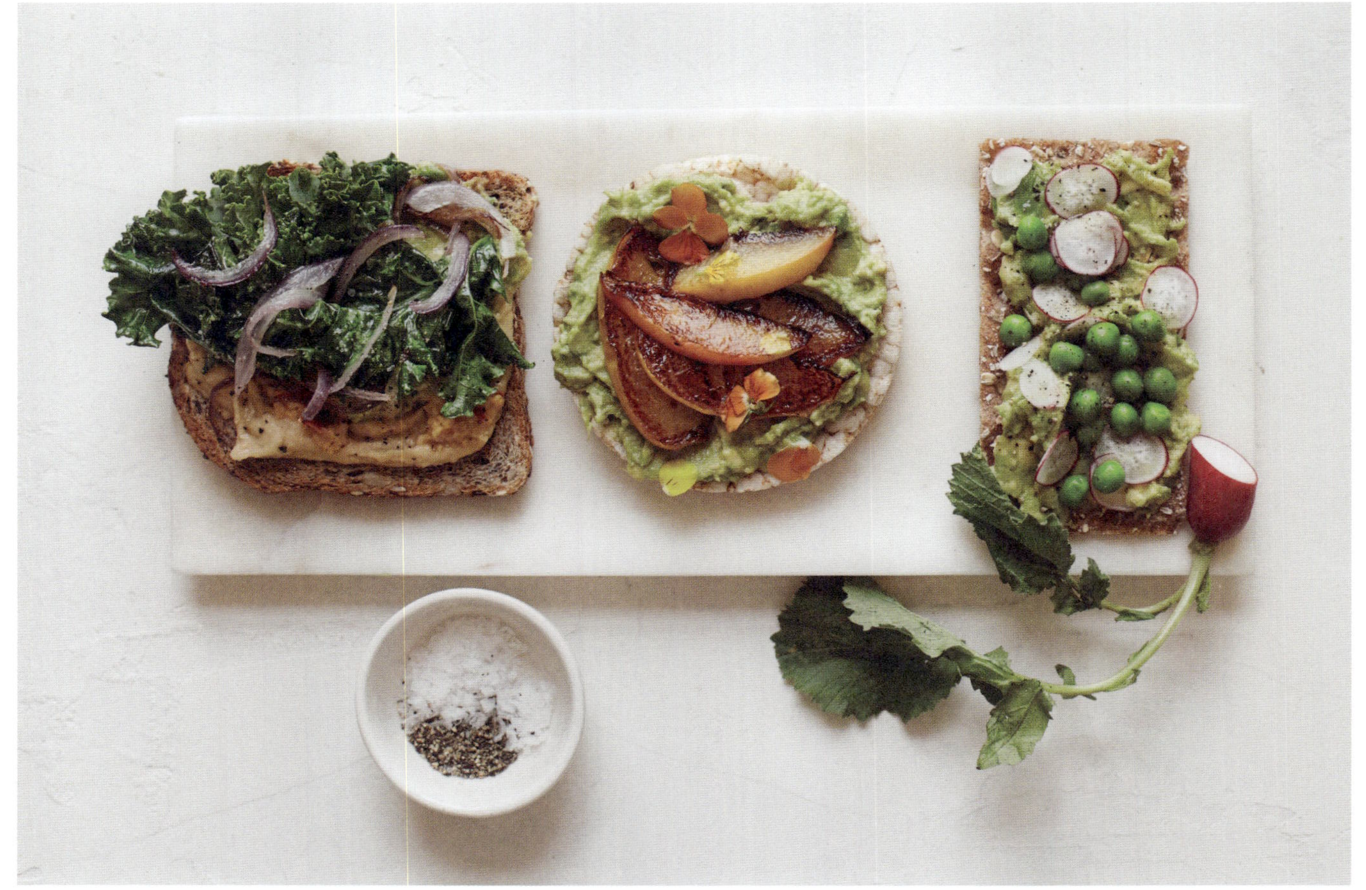

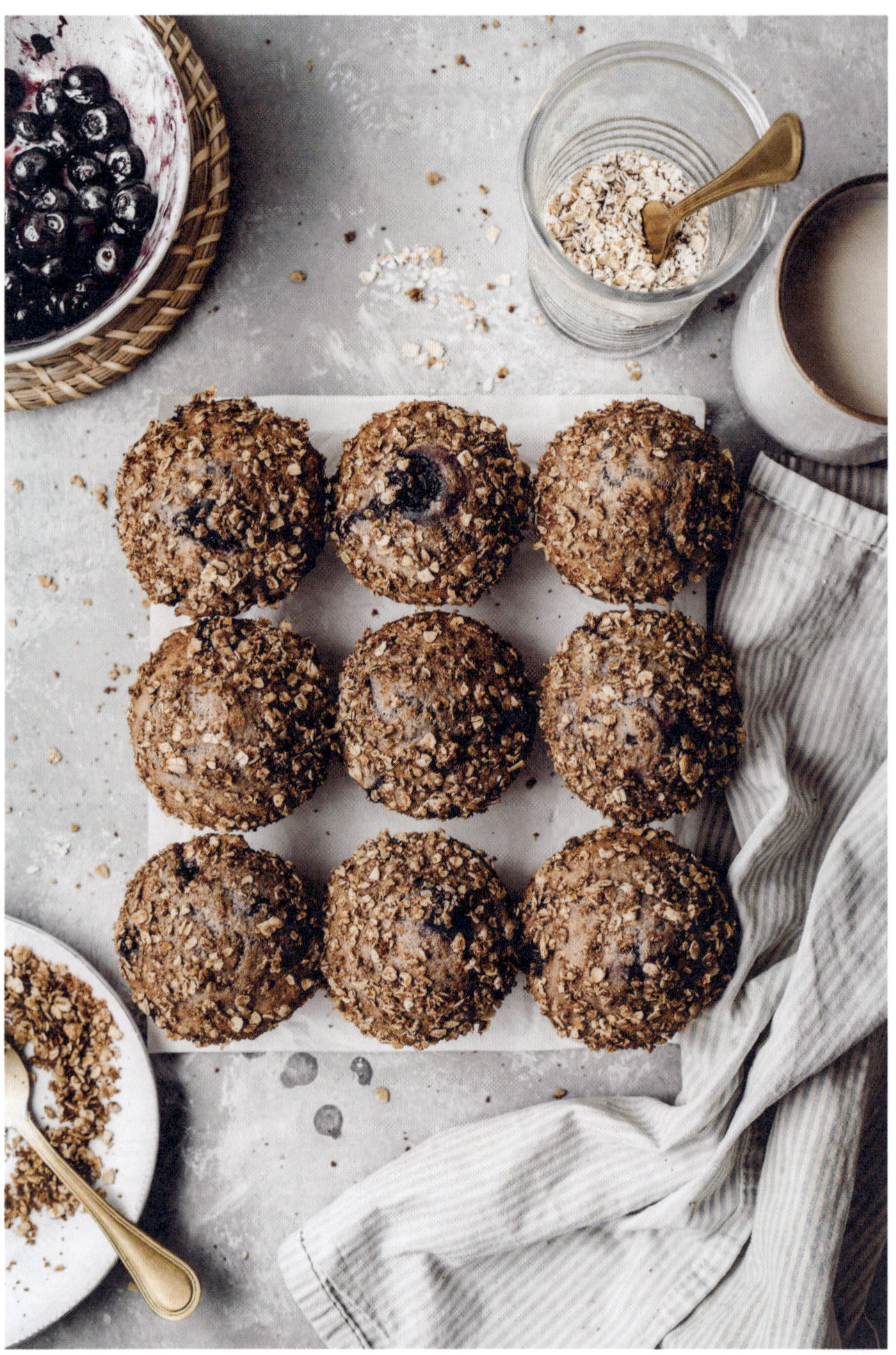

Blueberry Oat Muffins

When we honor what we do well, we can bring that competent energy and outlook to the areas in our life we are struggling with. The same transference principle applies in the kitchen. This muffin recipe happens to be one I always turn to when I'm in need of a little kitchen mojo-boost because it comes out amazing every time and tastes heavenly.

YIELD: 12 muffins

Coconut oil cooking spray, for greasing (or use paper baking cups)
2 teaspoons flaxseed meal
2 tablespoons (30 ml) water
½ cup (120 ml) unsweetened almond milk
1 teaspoon apple cider vinegar
1 cup (244 g) unsweetened applesauce
½ cup (48 g) gluten-free rolled oats
1 cup (94 g) gluten-free oat bran
⅓ cup (80 ml) maple syrup
¼ cup (37 g) date sugar (maple or coconut sugar work as well)
¼ cup (48 g) raw extra-virgin coconut oil, melted
2 teaspoons baking soda
1 teaspoon vanilla extract
1 teaspoon almond extract
½ teaspoon sea salt
1 cup (150 g) fresh blueberries (or frozen and slightly thawed) tossed in gluten-free 1-to-1 flour

Preheat the oven to 375°F (190°C, or gas mark 5) and grease a 12-cup muffin pan with cooking spray or line with paper baking cups.

Mix together the flaxseed and water and set aside for 5 minutes, until thickened.

In a measuring cup, mix the almond milk and apple cider vinegar and set aside.

In a large mixing bowl, combine the flax seed and almond milk mixtures, and the remaining ingredients (except blueberries) and mix well. Lightly fold in the blueberries.

Pour the batter into the muffin cups, about two-thirds full.

Bake for 10 to 12 minutes, or until a toothpick inserted into the center of a muffin comes out clean. Remove from the oven and set aside to cool before serving.

Visualization for Transference

Sit in a comfortable position with your spine straight and your eyes closed and focus on your third-eye point. Take long, deep breaths and call to mind an area of your life where you are thriving. See how you operate in this area of your life. What beliefs and principles drive you? What kind of energy sustains you? How do you feel when making decisions? Next, call to mind an area of your life that you are currently having trouble with. Visualize yourself in different situations, bringing the same principles, beliefs, and energy to this area as the one in which you thrive. Allow this transference to sink in. When you are ready, take a deep breath in. Hold it to soak up your new confidence, then exhale and relax.

“

I honor what's working.

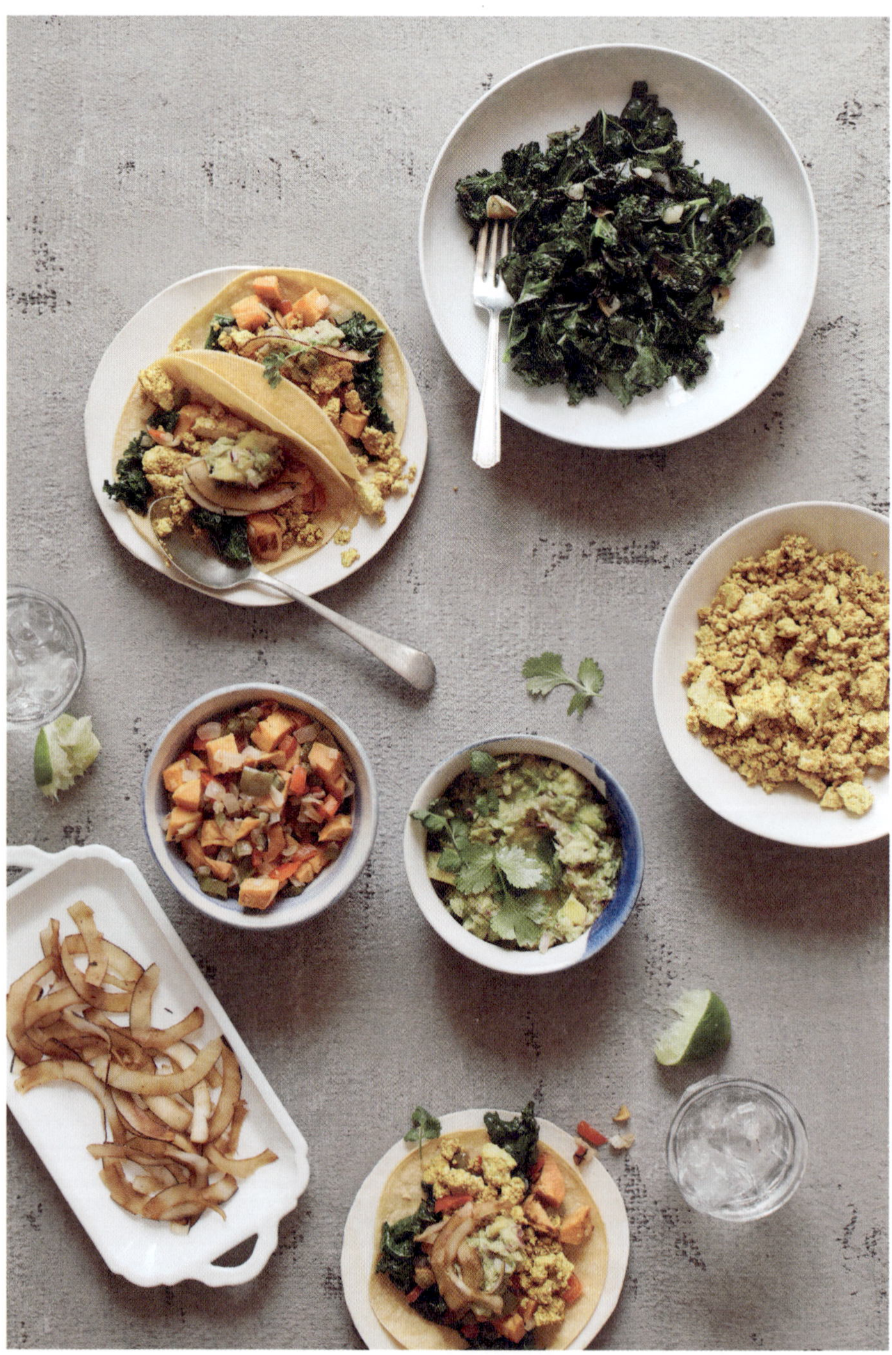

Brunch Tacos

Center yourself in gratitude for your abundance and watch it multiply. Nothing makes me feel more abundant than a meal made with lots of love—there's no meal I love more than brunch, and no food I love quite as much as tacos!

YIELD: 4 servings

HASH BROWNS

4 sweet potatoes, peeled and cut into 1-inch (2.5 cm) square chunks
1 white onion, diced
½ red pepper, diced
½ green pepper, diced
1 tablespoon (15 ml) extra-virgin olive oil
2 teaspoons garlic powder
2 teaspoons onion powder
1 teaspoon salt

MANGO GUACAMOLE

½ red onion, diced
1 tablespoon (1 g) chopped cilantro
2 ripe avocados, halved and pitted
1 mango, diced
Juice of ½ lime
½ teaspoon salt

TOFU SCRAMBLED "EGGS"

1 tablespoon (15 ml) extra-virgin olive oil
14-ounce (397 g) package extra-firm tofu, drained and crumbled
2 teaspoons ground cumin
2 teaspoons curry powder
2 teaspoons ground turmeric
2 teaspoons onion powder
2 teaspoons garlic powder

COCONUT BACON

½ cup (43 g) unsweetened coconut flakes
3 tablespoons (45 ml) tamari (gluten-free soy sauce)
1 tablespoon (15 ml) steak seasoning

SAUTÉED GREENS

3 cups (204 g) baby kale or baby spinach
1 clove garlic, chopped
1 tablespoon (15 ml) extra-virgin olive oil or sesame oil

TACOS

8 corn tortillas or gluten-free taco shells

PUMP UP THE PROTEIN:

Swap the coconut flakes for grilled tempeh, chopped up and tossed in the same sauce mixture, for an added protein punch. (Keep in mind the tofu already brings a solid amount of protein to the table!)

"

I appreciate my abundance.

To make the hash browns, preheat the oven to 425°F (220°C, or gas mark 7). In a medium mixing bowl, combine all the ingredients and toss well until thoroughly combined. Scatter the mixture onto a baking sheet and roast in the oven for 10 minutes, until browned and cooked through.

Meanwhile, to make the mango guacamole, toss the onion and cilantro in a medium bowl (or molcajete—the traditional Mexican version of the mortar and pestle) and press them into each other with the back of a spoon. In a separate bowl, lightly mash the avocado, then add it to the onion mixture along with the mango, lime juice, and salt. Mix well and set aside.

To make the tofu scrambled "eggs," heat the olive oil in a frying pan over medium heat. Add the tofu and spices and stir for 2 to 3 minutes until mixed through. Reduce to low heat while you complete the next steps.

To make the coconut bacon, combine all the ingredients in a small frying pan and spread out. Heat over medium heat and stir for 1 to 2 minutes, or until the coconut browns. Transfer the mixture to a small serving bowl.

Check on the hash browns, remove them from the oven, and set aside. Give the tofu scrambled eggs a good stir.

To make the sautéed greens, combine the baby kale or spinach, garlic, and olive oil in a medium frying pan and cook over medium heat for 3 to 5 minutes, or until the kale is bright green and wilted. Remove from the heat and place in a small bowl.

Place a tortilla in a dry frying pan over medium heat and cook for about 45 seconds on each side, until warm and lightly brown. Repeat with the remaining tortillas.

Serve all the components in separate bowls. My preferred assembly method starts with a generous helping of sautéed kale, a spoon of sweet potato hash, and topped with tofu scramble. Add a dollop of mango guacamole and a sprinkling of coconut bacon and there you have it—an incredible brunch treat!

Make Your Own Gratitude Meditation

Take out pen and paper, put on an upbeat playlist. Write down 100 things in your life you are grateful for. When you start running out of ideas, get creative. Include everything, from the big (being alive, the well-being of your family) to the small (the amazing book you're reading, the bird you spotted that made you smile). You have abundance in your life; allow it to flow out and be acknowledged—every last drop.

Once you've completed your list, hit the voice recorder on your phone and speak your entire list out loud. Save the recording as your personal gratitude practice; when you need to get back in touch with your abundance, find a comfortable place to sit, close your eyes, take a few deep breaths, and listen to your amazing gratitude inventory.

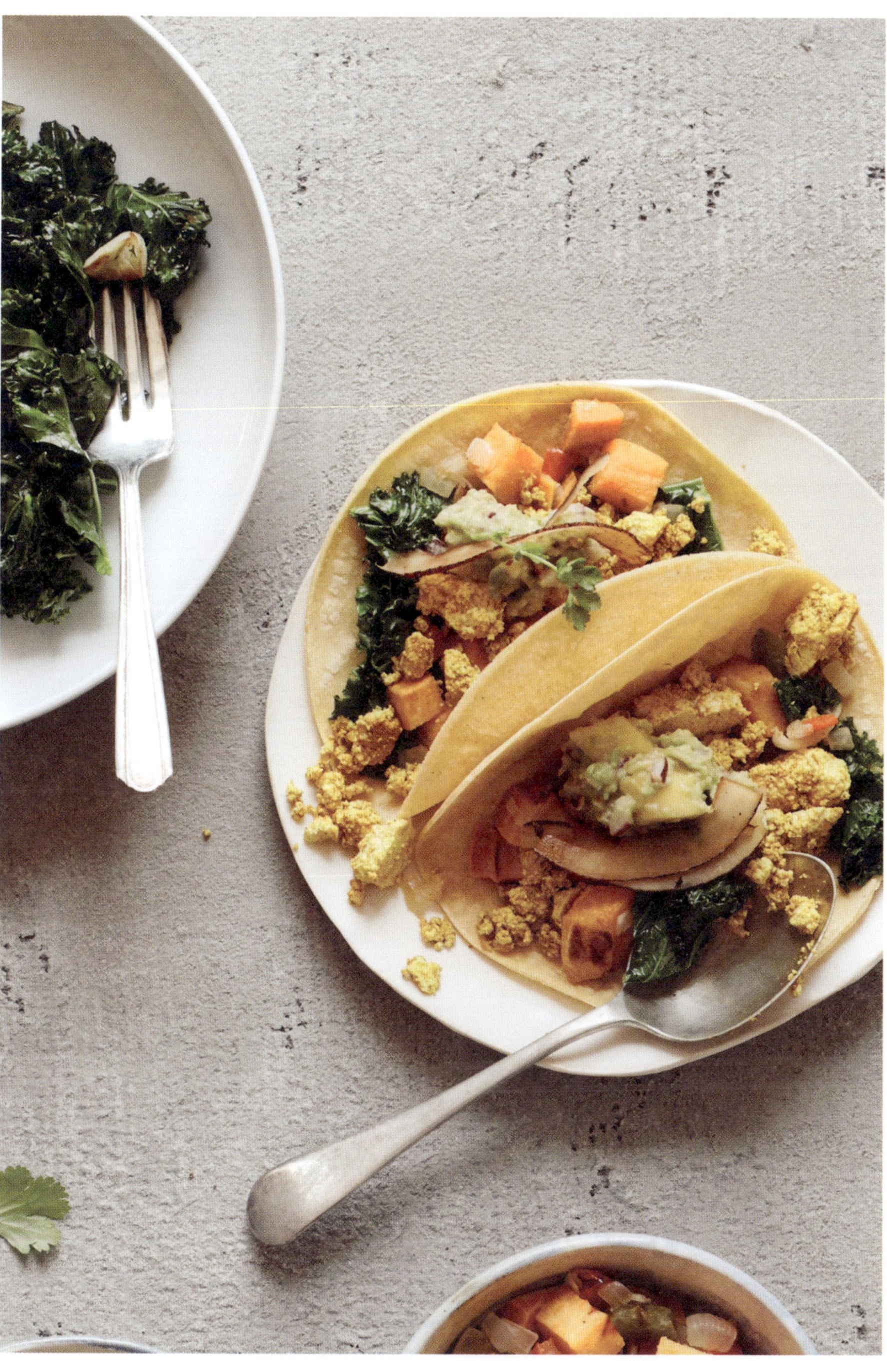

Chia Seed Pudding

Often when we are craving sweetness, especially first thing in the morning, it comes from a deep need to treat ourselves more "sweetly." This pudding was a very helpful breakfast, snack, and dessert for me when I was first transitioning off sugar. The vanilla, cinnamon, and berries are all truly nourishing ways to quiet that sweet craving.

YIELD: 1 serving (per option)

1 cup (240 ml) unsweetened vanilla coconut milk
⅓ cup (40 g) chia seeds
½ teaspoon vanilla extract
Pinch of ground cinnamon
Pinch of ground nutmeg
Pinch of ground cardamom
Fresh berries, to serve
Nuts, to serve

In a mason jar or a small bowl, combine the coconut milk with the chia seeds. Add in the vanilla, cinnamon, nutmeg, and cardamom. Mix and let sit in the refrigerator for an hour or until it reaches a pudding-like consistency. Stir periodically, if needed, to evenly distribute the chia seeds.

To serve, top with berries and nuts.

Self-Love Meditation

Light one of your favorite candles, put on a love song, and sit comfortably in a cozy spot in your home. Place your hands over your heart center, right on top of left. Feel the warmth and pulse of your heart as you close your eyes and take long, deep breaths. Feel a bright ball of golden light at your heart center, growing with each breath and creeping into every nook and cranny of your being. Enjoy this connection to the love you have within, perhaps even bringing to mind an image of yourself as a child. Feel yourself being held by your own loving energy as you would be held by a romantic partner. Stimulate that feeling from within and allow yourself to bask in your own warm, loving light.

When you are ready to release, take a deep breath in, allowing the light from your heart to form a big "love bubble" around you. Hold that breath for 15 seconds and then exhale, slowly bringing yourself back into the room.

"

My life is a reflection of how sweet I am to myself.

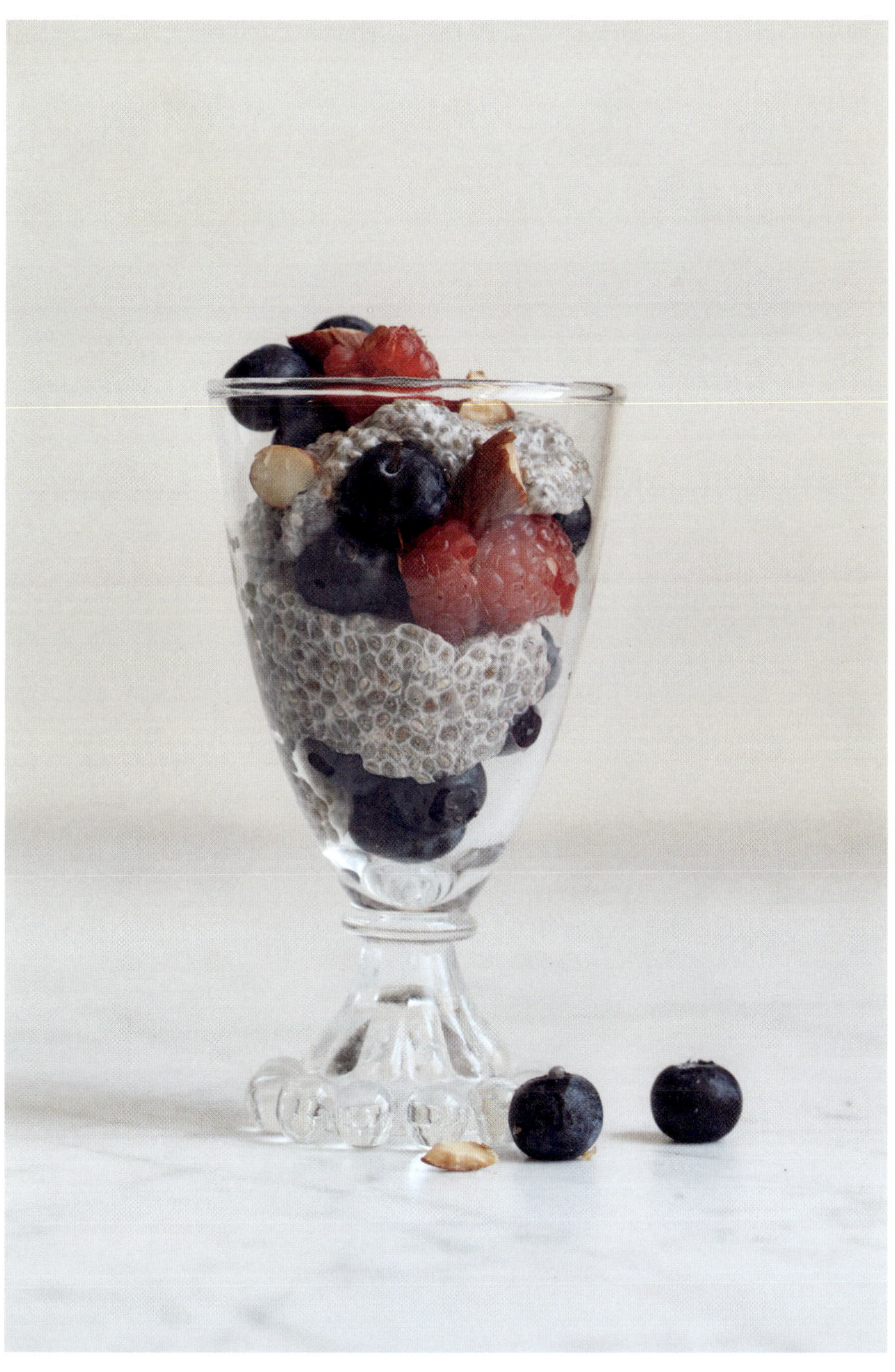

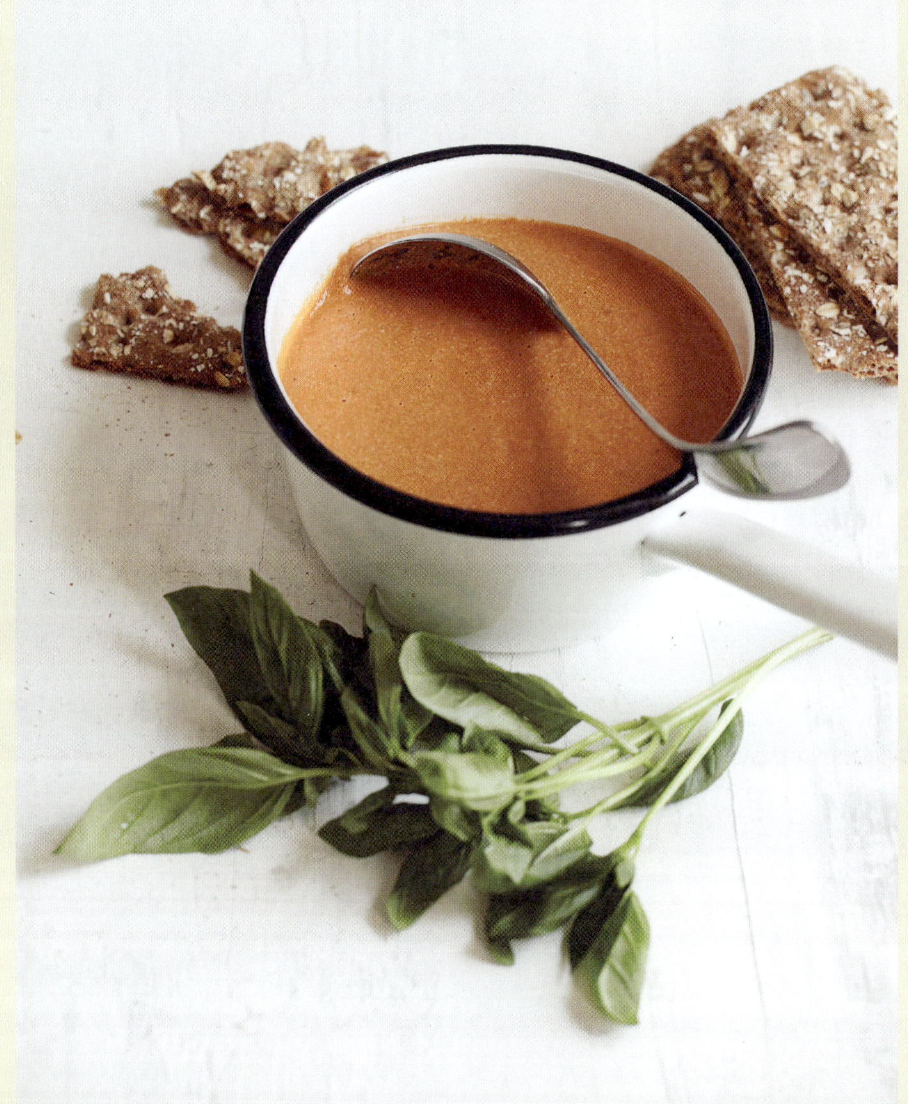

Creamy Tomato Soup

The only place you can ever find home is inside yourself—but some foods, like this creamy tomato soup, might help you call up that feeling of cozy belonging. Let the nostalgic flavors anchor you when you feel unmoored, and pair them with the meditation below when you are in need of balance. It's great for when you are worried, upset, or you're at a loss about what to do.

YIELD: 4 servings

2 tablespoons (30 ml) extra-virgin olive oil, divided
2 white onions, diced
1 clove garlic, chopped
½ cup (65 g) raw unsalted cashew nuts, soaked in water for 2 to 3 hours and drained
½ cup (120 ml) vegetable broth
(3) 14.5-ounce (411 g) cans stewed tomatoes
1 cup (240 ml) canned light coconut milk
1 teaspoon freshly ground black pepper
¾ teaspoon salt
½ teaspoon paprika
3 tablespoons (8 g) shredded basil leaves, to garnish

Heat 1 tablespoon (15 ml) olive oil in a large frying pan over medium heat. Add the onions and sauté for 5 minutes until softened, then add the garlic and sauté for another minute.

Transfer the mixture to a food processor or high-speed blender. Add the remaining 1 tablespoon (15 ml) olive oil, the soaked and drained cashews, vegetable broth, tomatoes, coconut milk, and spices and purée until thick and creamy.

Transfer the soup to a medium saucepan and heat over medium heat until the soup is warmed through. Serve hot and garnish with the basil leaves.

Kundalini Meditation for Emotional Balance

Before practicing this meditation, drink a glass of water. Sit comfortably and hug yourself, placing your palms open against your body, under your armpits. Raise your shoulders up tightly against your earlobes without cramping the neck muscles. Keep your spine straight and your chin gently tilted down in order to maintain the straight line of your spine. Close your eyes and allow your breath to slow naturally. Continue for 3 minutes, gradually building up to 11 minutes. To close the meditation, take a deep breath in, hold it, and then exhale to relax.

"

I am home.

Lentil Veggie Soup

When I assume the best of people and situations, it completely shifts my energy. I feel lighter and happier once I release the heavy burden of placing someone in the wrong. A hearty lentil veggie soup is a great, nourishing antidote to a blame-focused mentality, helping you ground yourself in that open-hearted energy.

YIELD: 4 servings

OPTION 1
15-ounce (425 g) can brown lentils, drained
1½ carrots, chopped
1 onion, diced
1 clove garlic, finely chopped
4 cups (960 ml) vegetable broth
2 cups (136 g) chopped kale or spinach
1 cup (145 g) peas
2 tablespoons (30 ml) extra-virgin olive oil
Salt and freshly ground black pepper, to taste

Put the lentils in a large bowl and pour in enough boiling water to cover them. Let sit for 15 minutes, and then drain.

Combine all the ingredients in a large saucepan over high heat. Bring to a boil, reduce the heat, and simmer for 5 to 7 minutes, or until the carrots and onions are cooked through. Season with salt and pepper. Serve.

Meditation for Seeing Innocence

Sit in a comfortable position with your palms facing up on your knees. Close your eyes and take long deep breaths. Bring the person about whom you are assuming the worst into your mind's forefront. Silently ask to see this person's innocence in the situation. Hold your gaze on them and allow the possible explanations for their actions to surface. Actively choose the thoughts that honor their pure goodness.

If you struggle with this, call to mind their child-self. See them in the pure innocence of their three- or five-year-old self. When you are ready, take a deep breath in and send a stream of love from your heart to theirs. Exhale, and come back into the room.

"

 I assume the best of people.

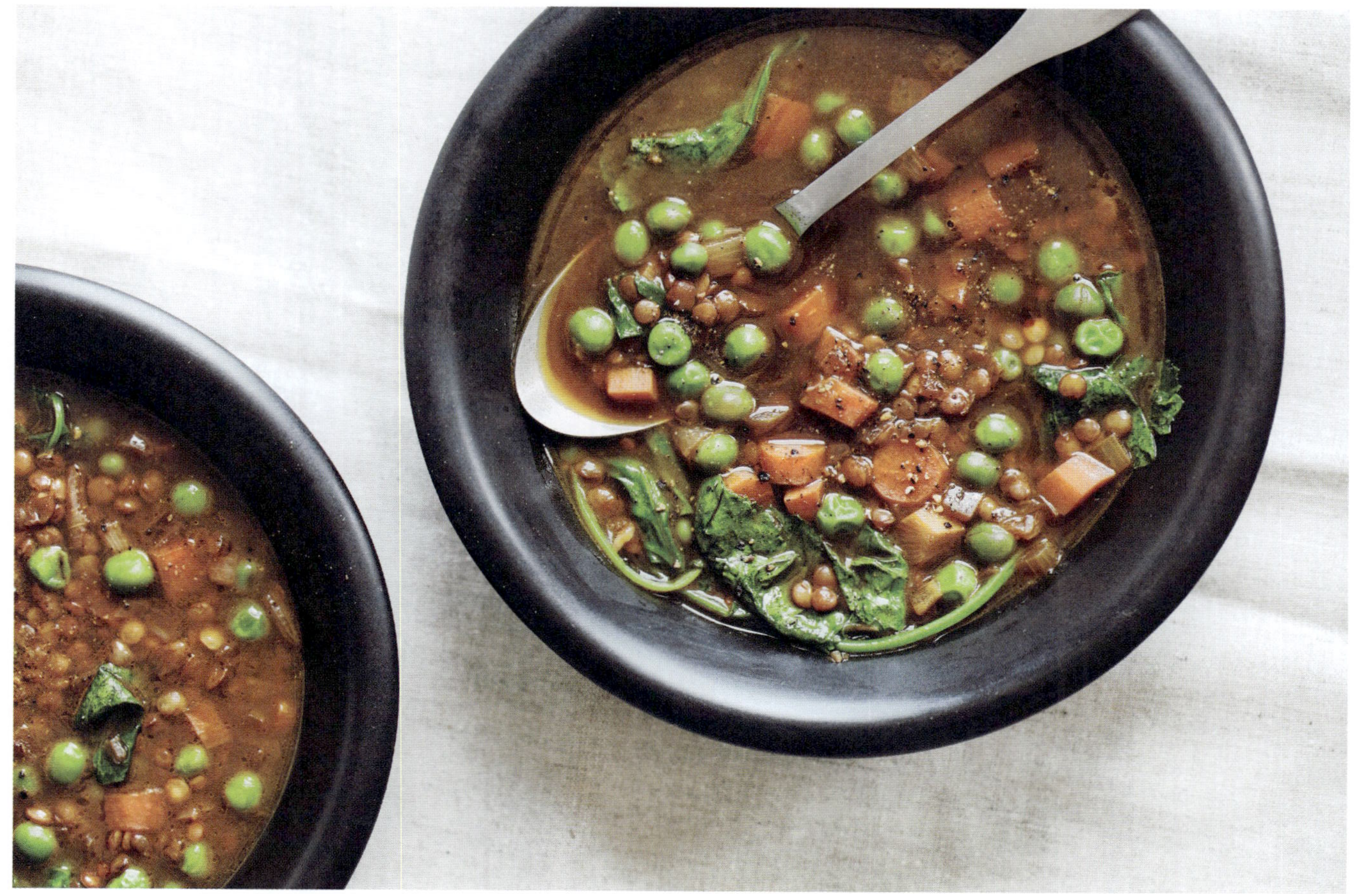

Spinach Artichoke Soup

You are the boss of your own life. When you call the shots, you can focus on the activities that help you be the best version of you. This savory, mouthwatering soup was inspired by my love of artichoke pizza—these days, I choose not to upset my body with gluten and dairy, but I still love eating flavorful, decadent food that makes me feel like a boss!

YIELD: 4 servings

1½ cups (170 g) canned or frozen artichoke hearts, thawed
1½ cups (45 g) spinach leaves
2 tablespoons (30 ml) extra-virgin olive oil
1 white onion, chopped
1 garlic clove, finely chopped
1 cup (240 ml) vegetable broth, divided
2 tablespoons (14 g) quinoa flour (or any flour you prefer)
1½ cups (360 ml) unsweetened almond milk
⅓ cup (20 g) nutritional yeast
2 tablespoons (30 ml) lemon juice
Pinch of salt
Pinch of freshly ground black pepper
2 scallions, thinly sliced lengthwise, to garnish

Put the artichoke hearts and spinach into a food processor and pulse until finely chopped. Set aside.

Heat the oil in a large saucepan over medium heat. Add the onion and sauté for 5 minutes until softened, then add the garlic and sauté for another minute. Pour in ½ cup (120 ml) vegetable broth, and then rapidly stir in the flour to form a smooth paste. Add the remaining broth and the almond milk and bring to a simmer.

Stir in the spinach and artichoke mixture, nutritional yeast, and lemon juice. Season with salt and pepper. Simmer for another minute, stirring continuously, until heated through.

Serve garnishedwith the scallion.

Stepping into your Boss Self

You can do this meditation seated or as a walking meditation.

Close your eyes and connect to your breath. Take a moment to plug into your own energy field and release any external noise. Call up an image of someone you admire who has powerful boss energy. Maybe it's Beyoncé, maybe it's your actual boss. Hold this inspirational figure in your mind and soak in their energy. If you are doing a walking meditation, open your eyes and keep them in soft focus on the path in front of you. Begin walking with this boss energy. If you are sitting, keep your eyes closed.

How would you approach the challenges or goals in your life right now with this powerful energy? How does this version of you organize your day? Mentally walk through a day in your life while you embody this energy. To close, allow every cell of your being to lock in this upgraded energy and take it with you as you move on with your day.

“

I am the boss of my own life.

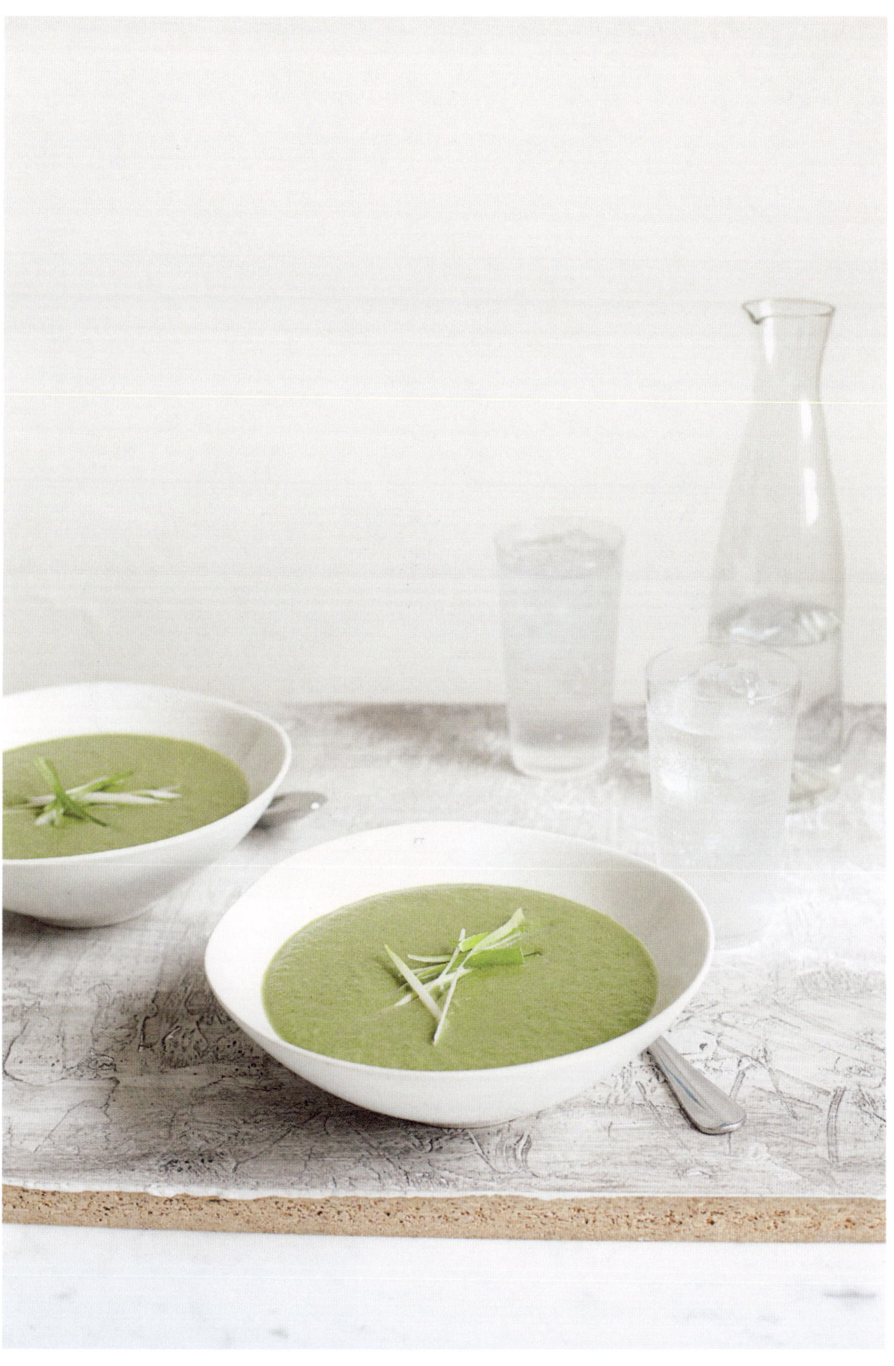

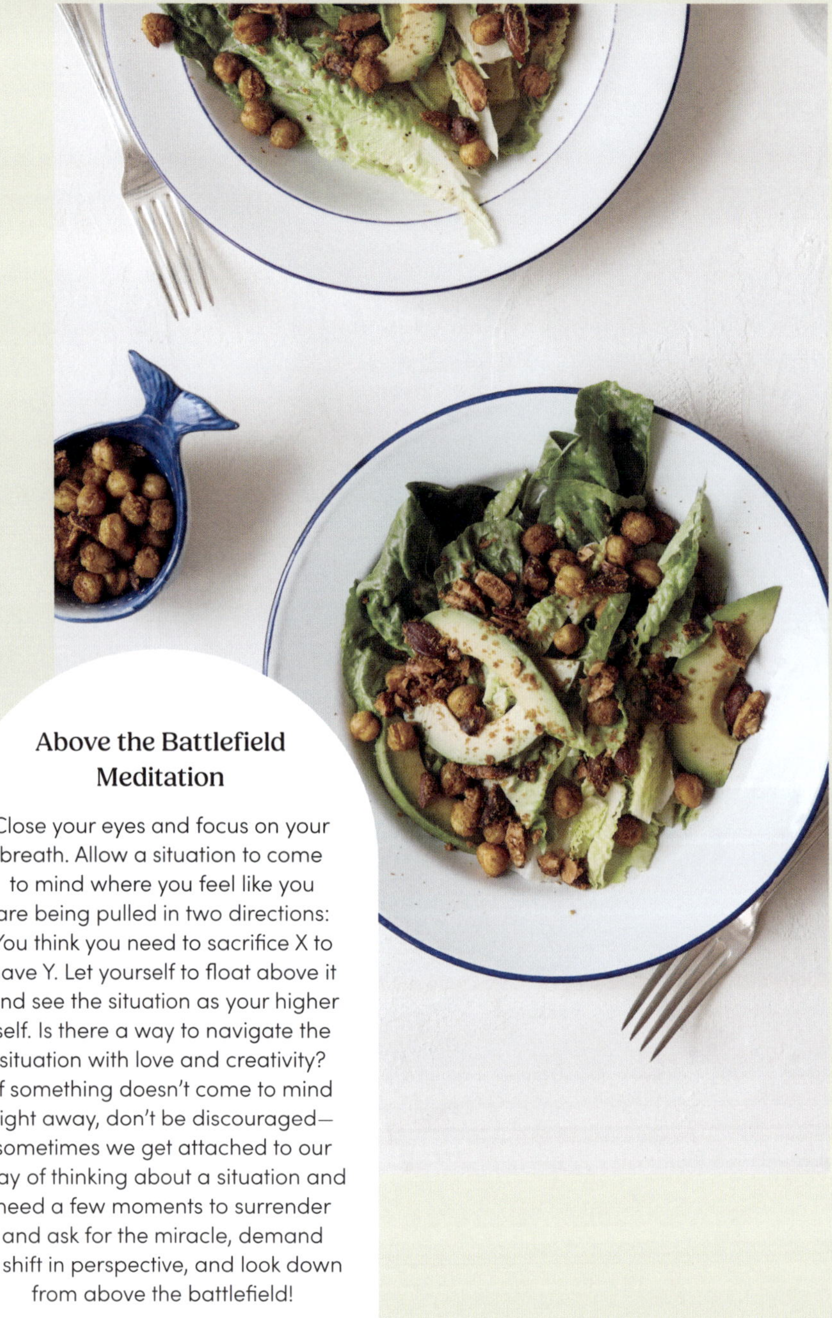

Above the Battlefield Meditation

Close your eyes and focus on your breath. Allow a situation to come to mind where you feel like you are being pulled in two directions: You think you need to sacrifice X to have Y. Let yourself to float above it and see the situation as your higher self. Is there a way to navigate the situation with love and creativity? If something doesn't come to mind right away, don't be discouraged—sometimes we get attached to our way of thinking about a situation and need a few moments to surrender and ask for the miracle, demand a shift in perspective, and look down from above the battlefield!

Caesar Salad

You may be faced with a situation where you feel like you need to choose between two things that are important to you. Allow yourself, for a minute, to hold the possibility of having the best of both worlds. When I first went vegan, I was upset about having to pass on my favorite Caesar salad. Once I gained a fresh perspective, I realized I could create the same textures and flavors using ingredients that I love!

YIELD: 2 servings

½ cup (82 g) precooked chickpeas, drained and rinsed
1 teaspoon extra-virgin olive oil, plus extra
2 teaspoons curry powder
1 teaspoon ground coriander
1 teaspoon ground turmeric
1 teaspoon garlic powder
1 tablespoon (15 g) nutritional yeast
Salt and freshly ground black pepper, to taste
4 ounces tempeh
1 teaspoon liquid smoke
1 teaspoon tamari
1 head romaine lettuce, leaves separated and coarsely chopped
½ red onion, quartered and sliced
1 avocado, halved, pitted, and sliced

DRESSING
1 tablespoon (15 g) garlic hummus
1 tablespoon (15 ml) extra-virgin olive oil
4 cloves garlic, crushed
Juice of ½ lemon
1 teaspoon dried oregano

Preheat the oven to 425°F (220°C, or gas mark 7). Line 2 baking sheets with parchment paper and set aside.

In a medium mixing bowl, combine the chickpeas, olive oil, curry powder, coriander, turmeric, garlic powder, nutritional yeast, salt, and pepper and toss until the chickpeas are thoroughly coated. Transfer the mixture to one of the prepared baking sheets and roast for 10 minutes, stirring occasionally, until they start to brown.

Meanwhile, slice the tempeh into thin 3-inch pieces and toss in a bowl with liquid smoke and tamari to marinate. Spread the tempeh slices on the second prepared baking sheet. Roast in the oven for 7 to 9 minutes, or until browned.

To make the dressing, combine all the ingredients in a small bowl and whisk until creamy. Season with salt and pepper.

Put the chopped lettuce and sliced red onion in a salad bowl, add the dressing, and toss lightly. Top with the roasted tempeh, chickpeas, and sliced avocado. Serve.

"

It's possible to have the best of both worlds.

Tofu Kale Waldorf Salad

This salad recipe came from my desire to make "body-friendly" versions of dishes I loved. Ultimately, loving and accepting your body helps you take better care of it. It helps you honor what feels good on a deep, nurturing level.

YIELD: 4 servings

2 tablespoons (30 ml) extra-virgin olive oil
16-ounce (454 g) package firm tofu, drained and cut into 3-inch (7.5 cm) cubes
⅓ cup (80 g) Dijon mustard
2 tablespoons (18 g) garlic powder
Salt and freshly ground black pepper, to taste
4 cups (272 g) chopped kale
1 Granny Smith apple, very thinly sliced
1 cup (151 g) sliced grapes
½ cup (51 g) chopped walnuts

DRESSING
16 ounces (452 g) dairy-free coconut yogurt
¼ cup (15 g) finely chopped fresh parsley
½ teaspoon ground oregano
Salt and freshly ground black pepper, to taste
Juice of 2 lemons

To make the dressing, combine the yogurt, parsley, oregano, and salt and pepper, and mix well. Stir in the lemon juice. Set aside.

Heat the oil in a medium frying pan over medium heat. Add the tofu, mustard, garlic powder, salt, and pepper and cook for 5 to 7 minutes, stirring occasionally. Reduce the heat to low and continue to cook while you prepare the rest of the salad (keeping an eye on the pan throughout).

Put the kale and dressing in a large bowl and massage the dressing into the leaves for a few minutes. (This softens the kale and distributes the dressing evenly!) Add the sliced apples, grapes, and walnuts.

Add the tofu to the salad mixture and toss. Serve.

Body Love Meditation

Find a comfortable place and sit or lie down. Close your eyes. Take long, deep breaths and allow yourself to be present in your body. Sit in gratitude for being alive, for having the opportunity to do the beautiful work you came here to do. Center on your heart. Feel it beating and sit in immense gratitude for the blood it pumps through your body, for its constant beating without any help from you. Now fill yourself up with gratitude for the following parts of your body one by one, as you did with your heart: your respiratory system; your nervous system; your skin, muscles, and skeleton; your blood; your digestive system; your reproductive system; and your endocrine system. Allow yourself to be saturated in the deep love and gratitude you have for your body in this moment. Take a deep breath in, hold it as you absorb that love and exhale.

"

My health is my greatest wealth.

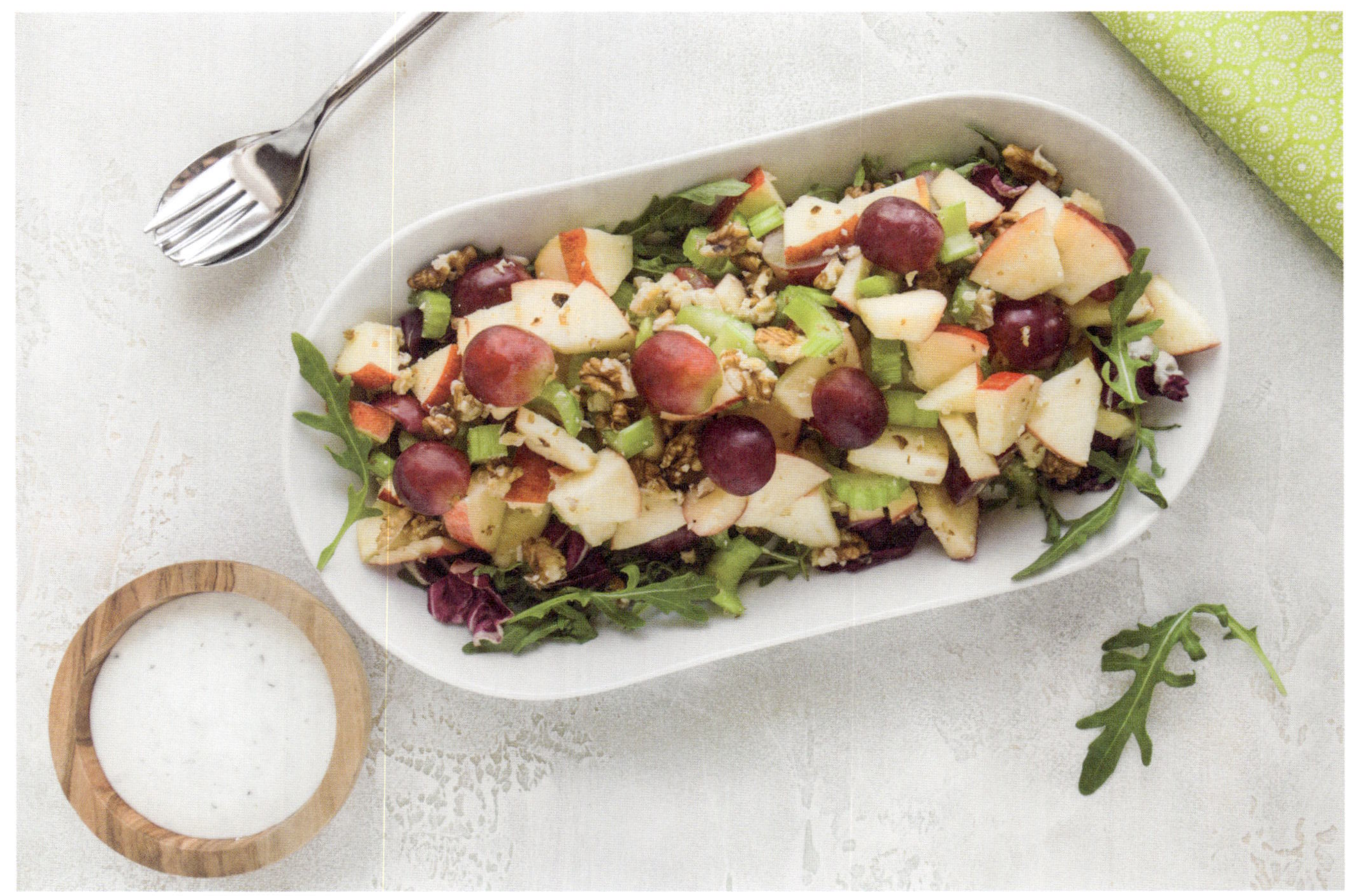

Taco Salad with Chili-Lime Ranch Dressing

Your power when handling any situation comes from your inner peace, so use this short and simple meditation to bring you back home in moments of frustration. One of the areas where I needed peace was in the kitchen, so I started small, making easy and accessible meals, and then slowly built up my kitchen mojo and got a little more creative.

YIELD: 2 servings

¼ cup (41 g) precooked chickpeas, drained and rinsed
½ cup (51 g) walnuts
2 tablespoons (30 ml) extra-virgin olive oil
1 teaspoon flaxseed meal
½ teaspoon ground cumin
½ teaspoon ground coriander
½ teaspoon paprika
½ teaspoon chili powder
½ teaspoon garlic powder
½ teaspoon onion powder
Salt and freshly ground black pepper, to taste
½ tomato, chopped
½ white onion, diced
¼ cup (4 g) chopped cilantro
1 jalapeño, chopped and divided
6 romaine lettuce leaves, chopped
½ cup (97 g) precooked black beans, drained and rinsed
1 avocado, halved, pitted, and sliced

“

My inner peace creates peace in the world around me.

CHILI-LIME RANCH DRESSING

¼ cup (60 g) tofu sour cream (this can be substituted with homemade cashew sour cream: prepare the Creamy Cashew Yogurt recipe on page 93 and add more lemon juice, to taste)
Juice from ¼ lime
Pinch of onion powder
Pinch of parsley
Pinch of garlic powder
Pinch of chili powder
½ teaspoon plain unsweetened almond milk

In a food processor, combine the chickpeas, walnuts, olive oil, flaxseed meal, cumin, coriander, paprika, chili powder, garlic powder, and onion powder. Generously season with salt and pepper and pulse until the mixture has the consistency of chopped meat. Set aside.

In a small bowl, combine the tomatoes, onion, cilantro, and a teaspoon of jalapeño and toss together.

Place the chopped romaine lettuce into 2 individual serving bowls. To each bowl, add ¼ cup black beans, half the tomato mixture, half the chopped "meat," and half the sliced avocado.

To make the chili-lime ranch dressing, combine all the ingredients in a bowl, mix together, and drizzle over salad.

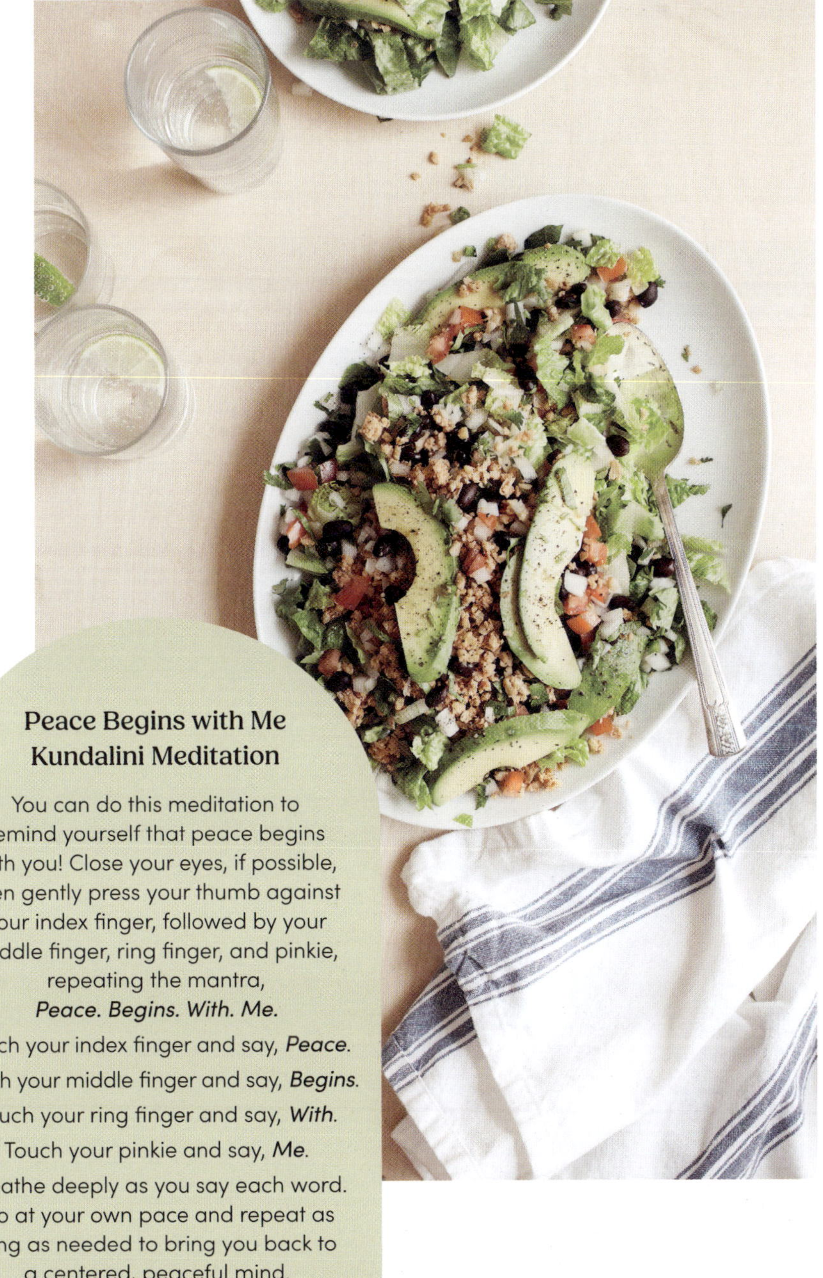

Peace Begins with Me Kundalini Meditation

You can do this meditation to remind yourself that peace begins with you! Close your eyes, if possible, then gently press your thumb against your index finger, followed by your middle finger, ring finger, and pinkie, repeating the mantra, ***Peace. Begins. With. Me.***

Touch your index finger and say, ***Peace.***

Touch your middle finger and say, ***Begins.***

Touch your ring finger and say, ***With.***

Touch your pinkie and say, ***Me.***

Breathe deeply as you say each word. Go at your own pace and repeat as long as needed to bring you back to a centered, peaceful mind.

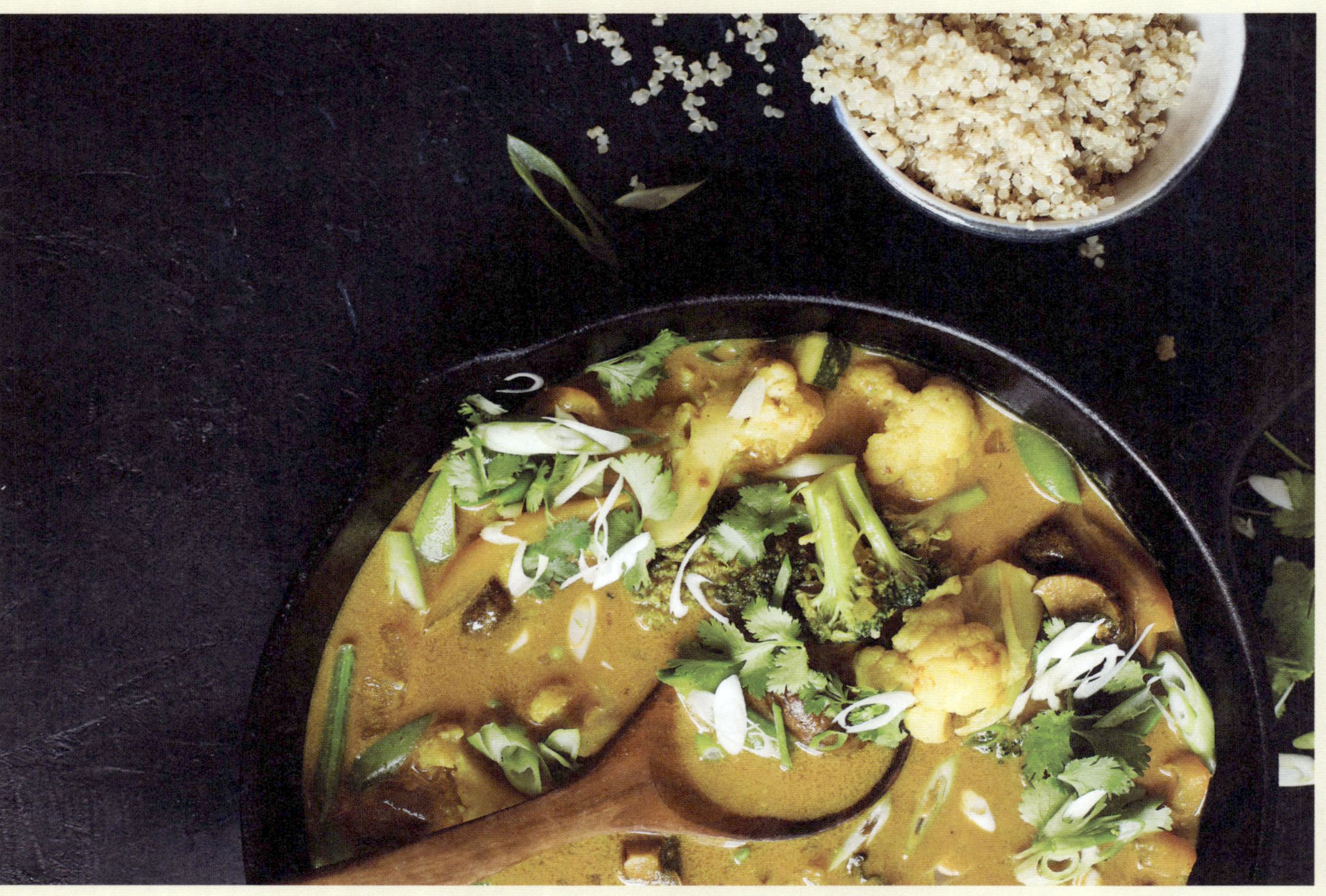

Veggie Curry

That thing that's getting in your way, those habits that are holding you back, that relationship that isn't supporting your growth: Let. It. All. Go. This dish is both nourishing and grounding, helping to center you so that you can move forward with conviction.

YIELD: 4 servings

1 tablespoon (12 g) raw extra-virgin coconut oil
1 white onion, diced
1 clove garlic, finely chopped
1 tablespoon (6 g) freshly grated ginger
2 tablespoons (34 g) curry powder
1 teaspoon ground cumin
1 teaspoon ground coriander
1 teaspoon ground turmeric
Pinch of ground cayenne pepper
½ cup (50 g) diced broccoli florets
½ cup (50 g) diced cauliflower florets
¼ cup (31 g) sliced carrots
(2) 14-ounce (403 ml) cans light coconut milk
1 cup (240 ml) vegetable stock
¼ cup (25 g) coarsely chopped snow peas
Sea salt and freshly ground black pepper, to taste
Chopped cilantro and scallion, to garnish (optional)
Warm naan bread, cooked quinoa, or steamed brown rice, to serve (optional)

Heat the oil in a large saucepan over medium heat. Add the onions and sauté for 5 minutes until softened, then add the garlic and sauté for another minute. Add the ginger and spices and stir for 2 to 3 minutes.

Add the broccoli, cauliflower, and carrots, and sauté for another 5 minutes. Pour in the coconut milk and vegetable stock, bring to a boil, reduce the heat, and simmer for 5 to 10 minutes. Add the snow peas and then simmer for another 5 minutes, until the vegetables are cooked through. Season with salt and pepper.

Transfer the curry to a bowl, garnish with cilantro and scallion, and serve with naan bread, quinoa, or brown rice.

Ships Setting Sail Visualization

Sit comfortably with your eyes closed and palms facing up, taking long, deep breaths. Release any tension and center on your breath. Now, envision yourself sitting on the edge of a long dock, looking out onto a beautiful lake. To your left, you see several small wooden boats, no bigger than a man's shoe. Pick up a boat and set an intention to release something you are ready to let go of. Hold the boat in your hands, bring this intention to mind, inhale, and as you exhale, drop your boat into the lake and watch it float away. Repeat this for the rest of your boats. When you are done, inhale deeply and sit in the sensation of lightness. Feel the relief from letting go of whatever was holding you back. Exhale and relax.

"

I release everything that is not serving me.

Lavender Tea Cookies

When you're ready to call something into your life, being in the space to relax and receive it is powerful. I love the idea of a lavender tea cookie that's delicate, sweet, and calming. It evokes the magnetic power of just *being* rather than *doing*.

YIELD: 12 cookies

1 cup (224 g) soy-free vegan butter, softened
1¼ cups (193 g) date sugar
¾ cup (180 ml) nondairy milk (such as coconut milk or almond milk)
2 tablespoons (30 ml) chopped fresh lavender (or 8 to 10 drops lavender essential oil)
1½ teaspoons vanilla extract
2 ⅓ cups (261 g) quinoa flour
¼ cup (32 g) cornstarch
1 teaspoon cream of tartar
½ teaspoon baking soda
¼ teaspoon salt
Lavender-colored sugar or crushed lavender flowers (optional)

In a large bowl, cream the vegan butter and sugar together for 2 to 3 minutes, until light and fluffy. Add the nondairy milk, lavender, and vanilla extract and mix well. Sift in the flour, cornstarch, cream of tartar, baking soda, and salt and mix until a soft dough forms. Cover the bowl and put it in the refrigerator and chill the dough for at least 30 minutes.

Preheat the oven to 350°F (180°C, or gas mark 4) and line a baking sheet with parchment paper.

Roll the dough into 12 equal-sized balls and place them 2 inches (5 cm) apart on the prepared baking sheet. Bake for 10 to 12 minutes, or until the cookies turn golden brown around the edges. Roll in lavender-colored sugar, if desired.

GET CREATIVE:
You can make these tea cookies in different flavors by swapping out the lavender oil and dried flowers for rose or jasmine. You can even go savory, using sage or rosemary for a unique twist. Like a more neutral tea cookie? Skip the flavor entirely!

Kundalini Adi Shakti Mantra

In Kundalini yoga, we use this mantra to connect with the divine feminine. If you are new to chanting mantra, you can start by simply playing a recording while you sit with your eyes closed, and focus on your breath. If you want to chant along with the recording, even better. It is powerful to hear your own voice say the mantra, so chant loudly with it.

Adi Shakti, Adi Shakti, Adi Shakti, Namo Namo

Sarab Shakti, Sarab Shakti, Sarab Shakti, Namo Namo

Pritham Bhagvati, Pritham Bhagvati, Pritham Bhagvati, Namo Namo

Kundalini Mata Shakti, Mata Shakti, Namo Namo

"

I allow myself to relax and receive.

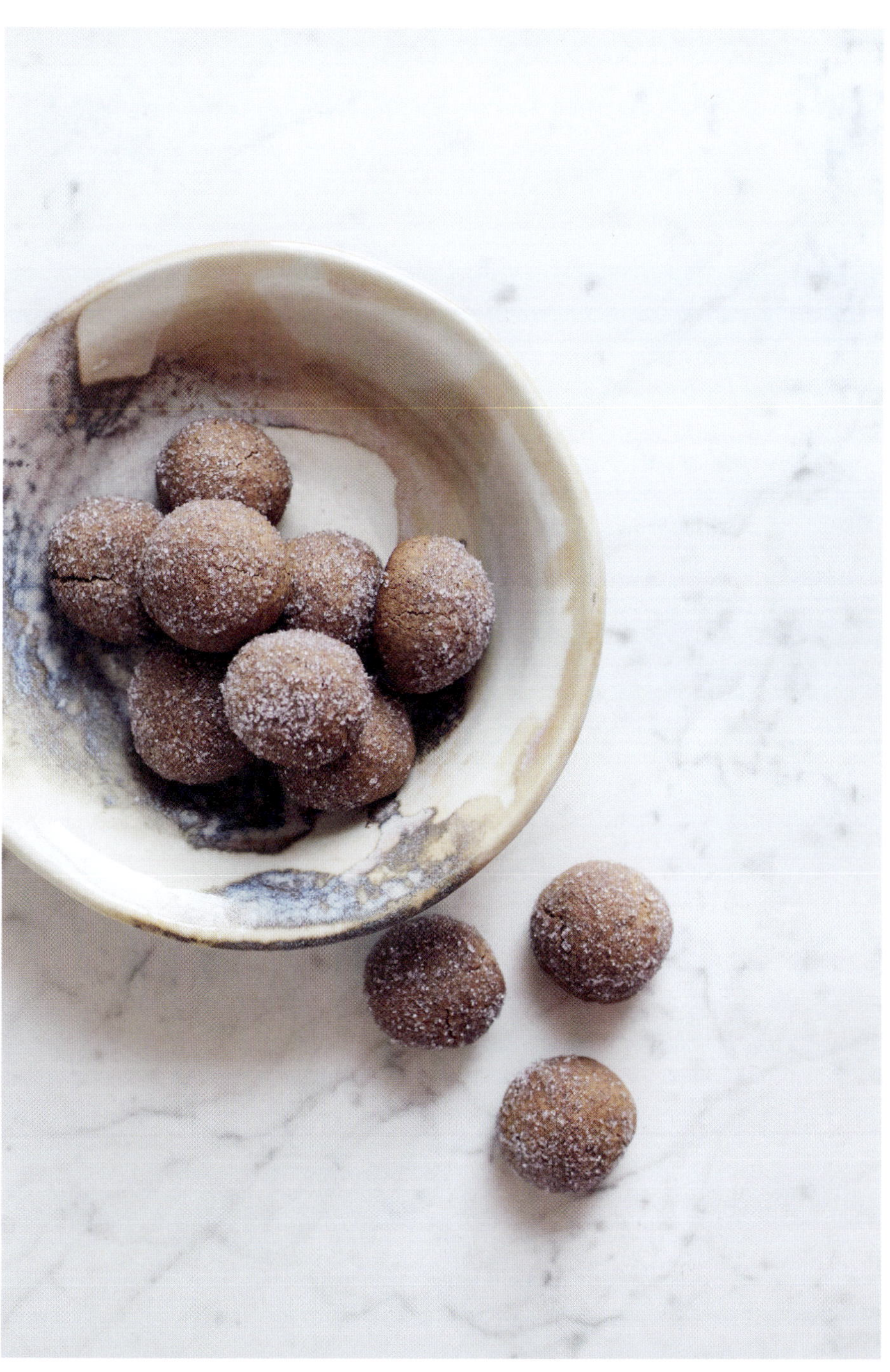

Mini Carrot Cakes with Cashew Cream Cheese Frosting

We are always leaning on something to find strength, whether it is faith, another person, or even fear. The good news is that you can shift back into your own knowing when you are reaching outside of yourself. When it comes to baking, I learned to lean on my soul early on. Whenever I make these carrot cakes, I am reminded to stay attuned to my magic.

YIELD: 12 mini cakes

CAKE

¼ cup (48 g) raw extra-virgin coconut oil, plus 1 tablespoon (12 g), for greasing (or use paper baking cups)
2 teaspoons flaxseed meal
2 tablespoons (30 ml) water
½ cup (120 ml) unsweetened almond milk
1 teaspoon apple cider vinegar
1 cup (244 g) unsweetened applesauce
1 cup (108 g) shredded carrots
1 teaspoon vanilla extract
1 teaspoon almond extract
¼ cup (54 g) date sugar (maple or coconut sugar work as well)
1 teaspoon baking soda
1 teaspoon baking powder
2 teaspoons ground cinnamon
1 teaspoon ground nutmeg
½ cup (51 g) chopped walnuts
1¼ cups (185 g) gluten-free 1-to-1 flour

ICING

1½ cups (195 g) cashew nuts, soaked in water for 2 to 3 hours and then drained
¼ cup (60 ml) canned coconut milk
¼ cup (22 g) unsweetened coconut flakes
4 teaspoons vanilla extract
Juice of 1 lemon
10 drops vanilla stevia

GARNISH

Pinch of ground cinnamon
Chopped walnuts, to taste

Preheat the oven to 375°F (190°C, or gas mark 5) and grease a 12-cup muffin pan with coconut oil or line with paper baking cups.

To make the cake, first make the flax "egg." Mix together the flaxseed and water in a small bowl and set aside for 5 minutes, until thickened.

Combine the almond milk and apple cider vinegar in a large measuring cup, stir, and set aside to curdle.

Combine the remaining cake ingredients in a food processor and pulse to combine. Add in the flax "egg" and almond milk mixture and purée until the consistency is like cake batter. Pour the mixture into your muffin cups, filling them halfway (and keeping the top flat for the icing). Bake for 15 minutes, or until a toothpick inserted into the center of the cake comes out clean. Set aside to cool.

To make the icing, combine all ingredients in a food processor or blender and mix well. Place the icing in the refrigerator to chill while the cakes are cooling. Give the icing a good stir before icing the cupcakes.

Garnish with cinnamon and walnuts.

"

I choose to lean on my soul.

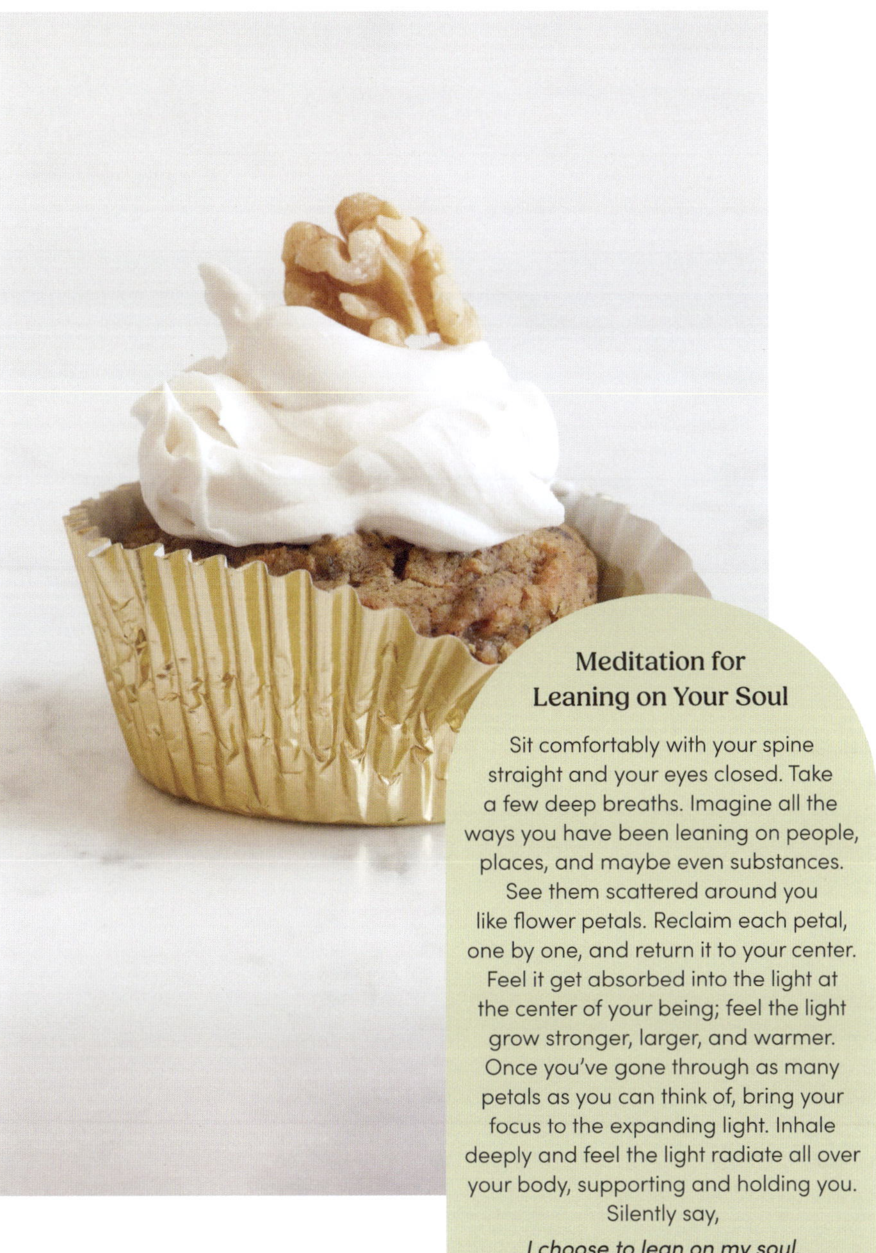

Meditation for Leaning on Your Soul

Sit comfortably with your spine straight and your eyes closed. Take a few deep breaths. Imagine all the ways you have been leaning on people, places, and maybe even substances. See them scattered around you like flower petals. Reclaim each petal, one by one, and return it to your center. Feel it get absorbed into the light at the center of your being; feel the light grow stronger, larger, and warmer. Once you've gone through as many petals as you can think of, bring your focus to the expanding light. Inhale deeply and feel the light radiate all over your body, supporting and holding you. Silently say,

I choose to lean on my soul.

Exhale and relax.

02

Summer

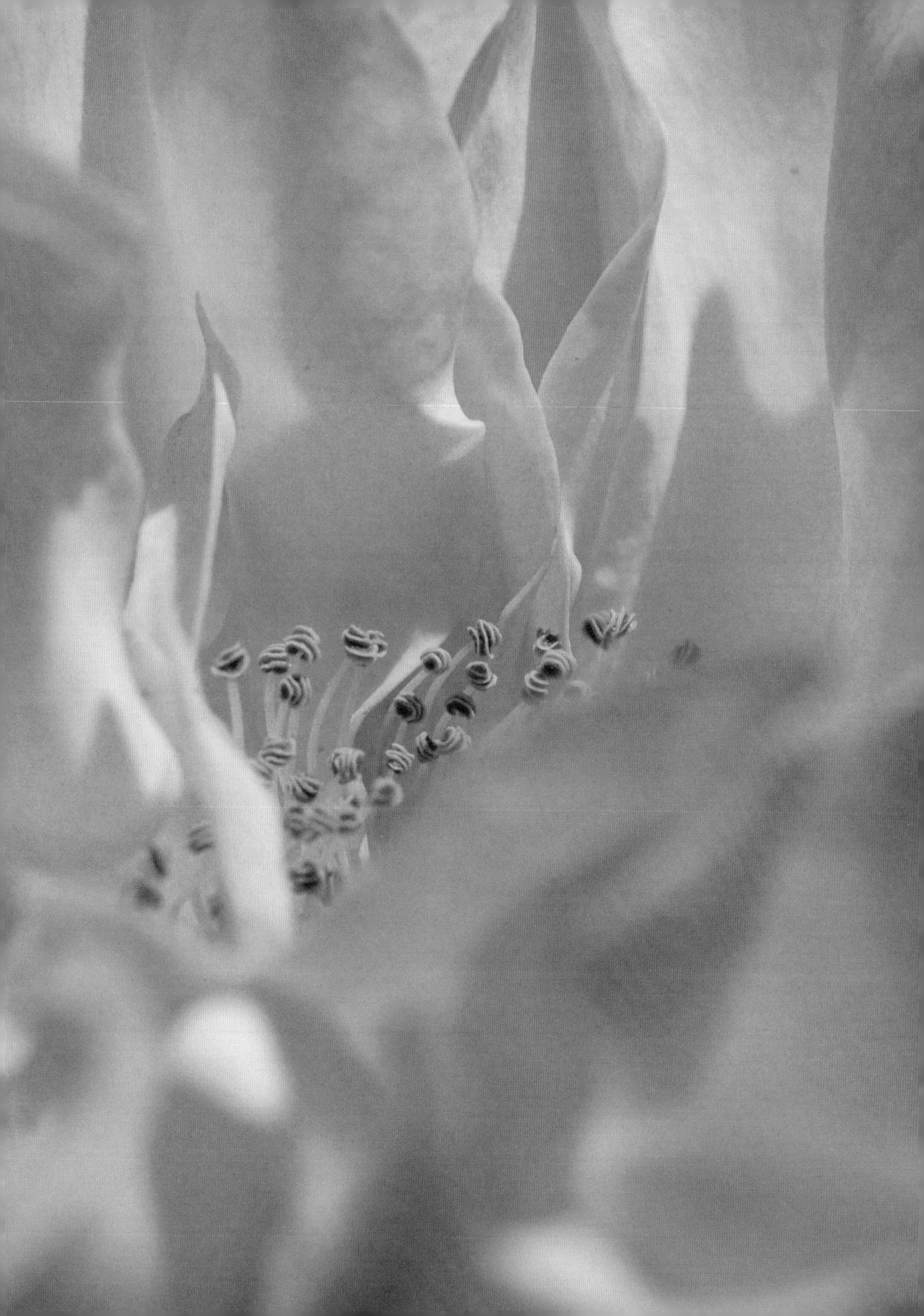

Blueberry Basil Juice

When we shift our attention from the "perceived problem" that is the cause of the stress to the sweetness all around us in each moment, we see things with greater clarity, allowing us to revel in our blissful, blessed lives! Drink this juice, soak up the sweetness of clarity in your life, and open up the portal for a clearer mind, body, and soul.

YIELD: 1 serving

5 sprigs basil
2 cups (134 g) chopped kale or spinach
1 green apple, coarsely chopped
1 lemon, peeled
1 cup (150 g) blueberries
¼ cup (36 g) blackberries

Starting with the basil, juice all the ingredients into a large glass.

Lightly stir and serve immediately.

Sweet Moments Meditation

This meditation is a little different because it involves a series of little moments throughout the day. The intention is to get you into the practice of "savoring the sweetness" in your day-to-day life. Set hourly alarms on your phone for the day with the message "take a sweet moment" or "savor the sweetness" on each alert. As each alarm sounds, stop what you're doing and give yourself a full minute to take some deep breaths and recalibrate your mind to the sweetness of that moment. Allow yourself to be inspired by the first thing that pops into your mind, to be grateful for it, and to let that feeling permeate your being while the breath calms and centers you. Repeat as many times as necessary with the intention of integrating it into your every day.

"

I savor the sweetness in my life.

Green Lemonade

I used to drink endless lattes to get through the day and help me stay focused on my work. In reality, the sugar and caffeine were making me feel awful at the end of the day. When I decided to replace them with an alkalizing daily green juice and pranayama (breath work practice), I not only got my beautiful clarity and focus back but had my body feeling nourished as well.

YIELD: 1 serving

5 romaine lettuce leaves
3 lemons, peeled
1 cucumber, peeled
1 pear, coarsely chopped
1 cup (68 g) chopped kale or spinach

Juice all the ingredients into a large glass. Lightly stir and serve immediately.

"

I am clear and focused

Pranayama Energizer Series

Breath of Fire: Sit comfortably. Begin rapid and forceful breathing out your nose (as if you were blowing out a candle with your nose). Focus on the exhale and allow the inhale to come reflexively. Continue breathing for 3½ minutes, then inhale deeply and hold the breath for 10 seconds. Exhale and relax.

Long Deep Breathing: In the same pose, breathe in long, complete breaths. Breathe deeper than normal so that your entire rib cage is used and lifts several inches on the inhale. Exhale and pull your navel all the way back. Consciously follow each part of the breath. Continue for 2½ minutes, then inhale and hold for 10 seconds. Exhale and relax. Pucker your lips and immediately inhale deeply through them. Exhale through the nose. Continue for 90 seconds, then inhale, hold briefly, and exhale.

Breath of Fire: Repeat exercise 1. Make your breathing powerful and regular for 1 minute, then inhale deeply and hold, as you focus on your third-eye point (the space between your eyebrows). Exhale and relax.

Breath Awareness: Meditate on the flow of breath as you relax and your breath settles into a normal rhythm. Feel the subtle pathways of the breath throughout your body. Sense the different kinds of energy that flow through every organ and cell.

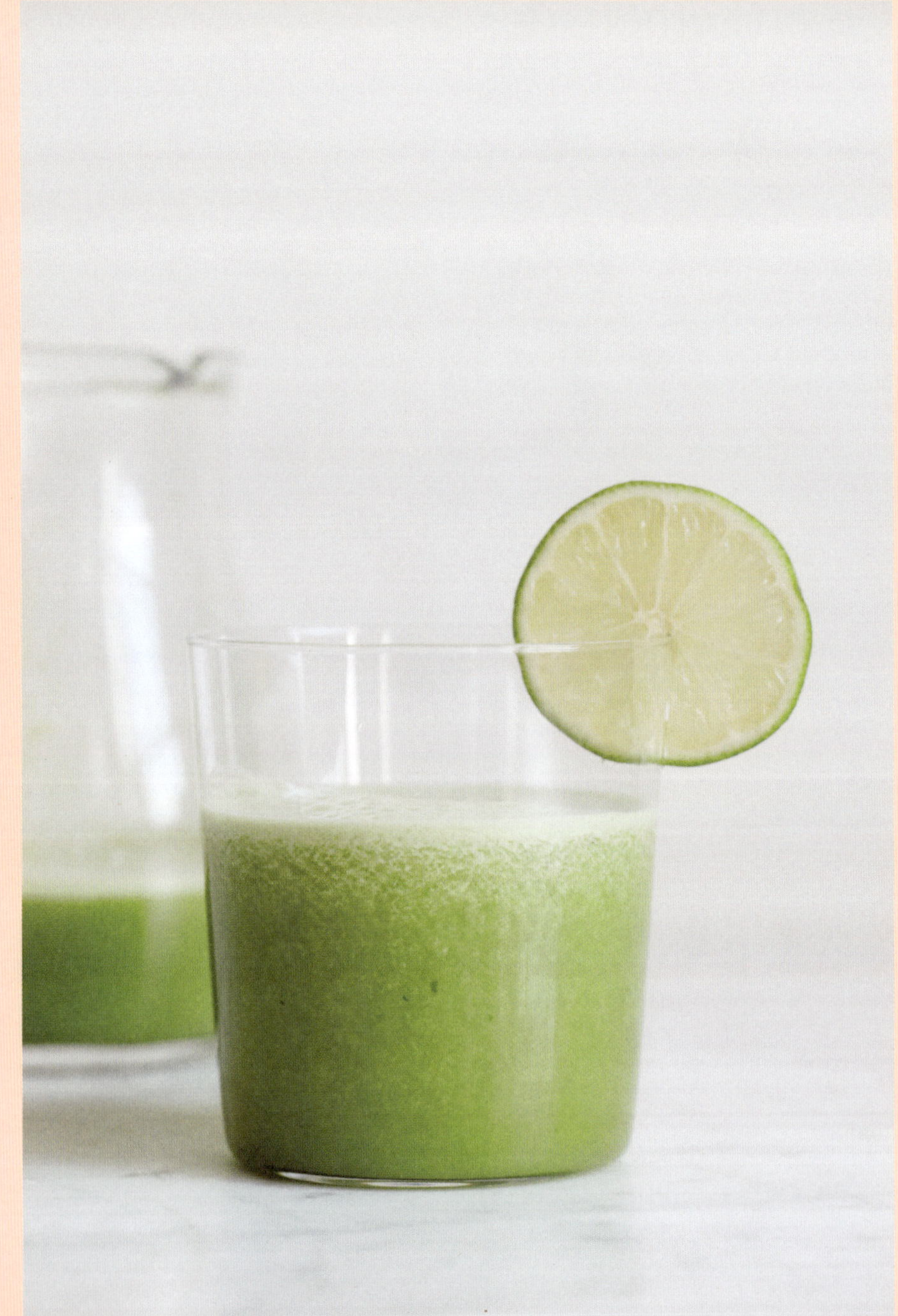

Radiance Juice

You can't fake true radiance. Thinking thoughts that nourish your soul and eating foods that nourish your body are more effective than the most luxurious makeup money can buy. This juice is packed with nutrients that will get you glowing from the inside out! Pineapple juice promotes healthy skin and helps prevent acne; watercress is great for your overall health with its high levels of vitamin C; and cucumber has cooling and moisturizing properties. In the paired exercise, we pull energy from our heart center and allow it to saturate every cell of our being, filling us with light and allowing our inner radiance to pour outward.

YIELD: 1 serving

½ cup (17 g) watercress (or romaine, if you can't find watercress)
2 cucumbers, peeled
2 limes, peeled
1 cup (166 g) pineapple chunks

Starting with the watercress, juice all the ingredients into a large glass.

Lightly stir and serve immediately.

Radiant Heart Meditation

Begin by sitting comfortably and breathing long and deep. Close your eyes and focus on your heart center while using your hands to slowly and steadily pull the energy surrounding you into your heart. Your hands should stay at heart height and move from the sides of your body inward, as if you are catching a ball and bringing it into your heart. Feel the light in your heart expand and grow brighter with each motion. Continue for at least 3 minutes, gradually building up to 11 minutes. Take a deep breath in and bring your hands into your heart, right palm on top of left. Feel the energy pulsing through your heart center and allow it to distribute throughout your entire being. Imagine it filling up each cell with loving energy. Exhale.

“

My beauty radiates from within.

Watermelon Mint Juice

This juice is always a special treat for me and feels like a rejuvenating island breeze at just the right time of the day. I love the balance of the watermelon with the cooling, alkalizing cucumber and refreshing mint. It's a great reminder that you can always call in a breeze or a peaceful rainfall to cool down and refresh your inner landscape. The paired breathing exercise will also leave you feeling cool, calm, and refreshed, and is a great daily practice.

YIELD: 1 serving

1 cucumber, peeled
1¼ cups (190 g) chopped watermelon
½ cup (15 g) fresh mint leaves
3 drops food-grade lavender essential oil (optional)

Juice the cucumber, watermelon, and mint into a large glass.

Lightly stir, add the lavender essential oil, if using, and serve immediately.

Sitali Pranayama (Cooling Breath)

Sit comfortably. Then touch your index finger to your thumb on each hand. (This is the gyan mudra.) Stick your tongue out and curl it up to form a taco-shell shape. If you can't curl your tongue, simply keep your tongue out and make an "O" shape with your mouth so that it naturally bends. Breathe in deeply through your tongue and mouth, allowing the air to fill you all the way up, then release through your nose. Repeat for 3 minutes, focusing on your breath and allowing yourself to enjoy the cooling sensation. To close, take a deep breath in, hold, and release.

"

I am refreshed and relaxed.

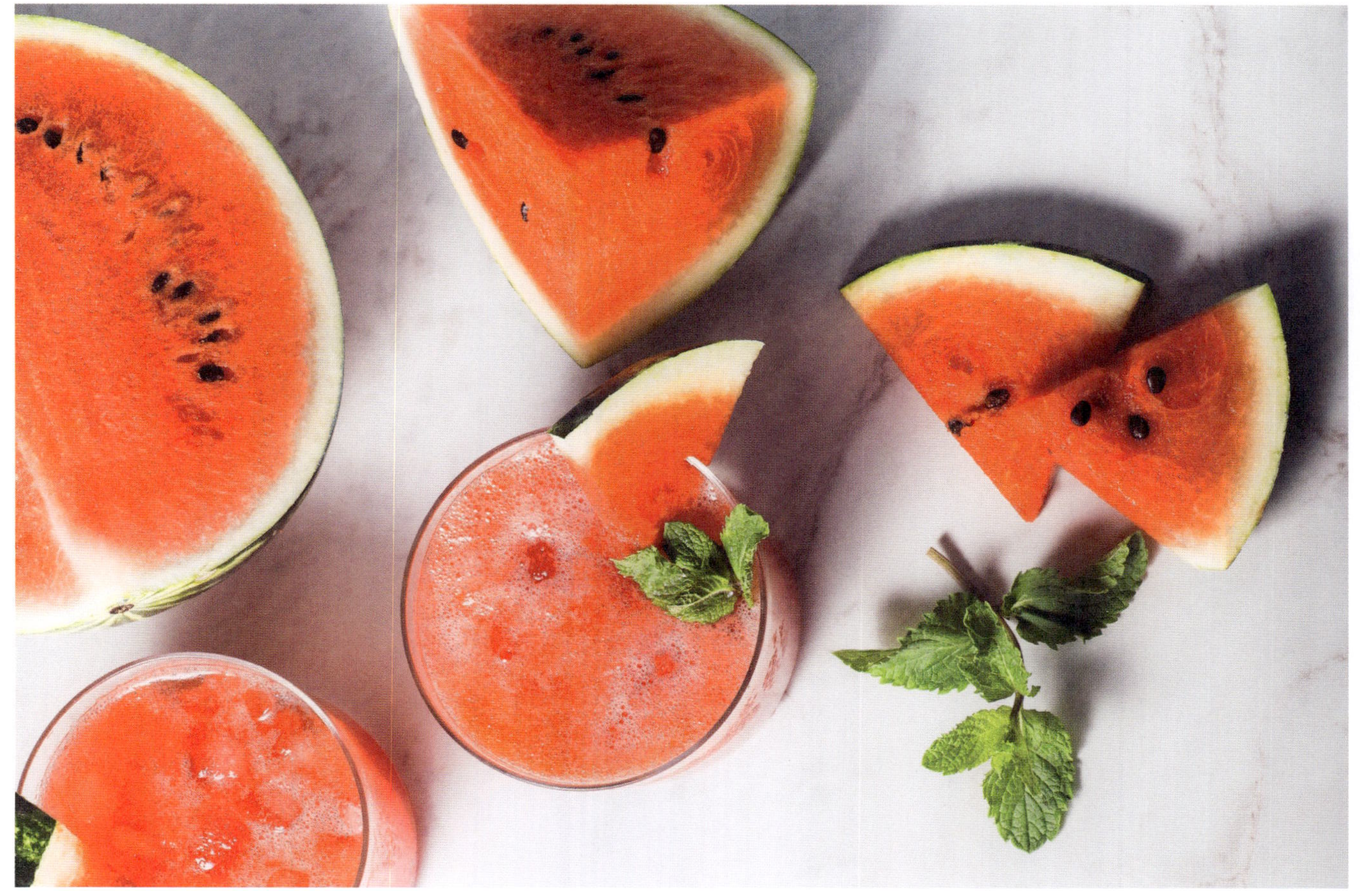

AB&C Protein Balls

Let. It. Be. Easy. Those four words have been a major game changer for me. What are you making "hard" or "difficult" in your life? This recipe is a simple yet nourishing breakfast that you can make ahead of time and grab on the go in a pinch for busy weeks when you just need it to be easy. I leaned on these *a lot* postpartum as a quick, filling snack I could grab throughout the day.

YIELD: 8 servings (1 serving = 3 balls)

3 cups (240 g) rolled oats
½ cup (60 g) plant-based protein powder of your choice
½ teaspoon ground cinnamon
2 teaspoons chia seeds
½ cup (125 ml) maple syrup
1 teaspoon vanilla extract
1 cup (256 g) nut butter of your choice (I love almond or cashew)
½ cup (80 g) dried cranberries

Combine the oats, protein powder, cinnamon, and chia seeds in a bowl. Mix until well combined and then add in your maple syrup, vanilla extract, and nut butter.

Mix together well and then fold in the dried cranberries. Grab a small piece of the dough and roll it in your hands to form a 3-inch ball.

Put a piece of waxed paper on a baking sheet and place your finished protein balls on top of it. Store in the fridge to firm them up and then grab them as needed.

GET CREATIVE:
This is a really easy recipe to play around and get creative with. Don't like cranberries? Swap for dried blueberries or cherries! Want a little chocolate treat? Use chocolate protein powder and toss in ½ cup of dairy-free chocolate chips instead of the cranberries. The possibilities are endless!

Waves of Abundance Meditation

This is a personal practice of mine. I do it at any time, in any position, whenever I feel frustrated or stuck. I'll sit on a park bench or pause while running errands and put on an uplifting song.

Close your eyes and imagine yourself standing in the middle of the ocean with beautiful, big waves gently rolling toward you. Allow yourself to sit in this powerful, natural flow of water and feel the waves of blessings on their way. After a few moments, envision yourself leaning back into the water and letting it support you as you float and soak in the rays of the sun. Allow this feeling to bring you back to your truth and remind you to enjoy the ease and flow of life.

"

I enjoy the ease and flow of life.

Chilled Protein Chia Oats

If we tell ourselves that our options are diminishing rather than expanding, we can't help but feel distressed. When we sit from a place of trust and turn our vision to the numerous possibilities before us, we naturally shift into a place of ease, flow, and peace. Chilled oats are a grounding treat that can put us in a calm state to see the possibilities ahead.

YIELD: 1 serving

1 cup (238 g) unsweetened vanilla coconut milk (or any dairy-free milk)
1 scoop of your favorite plant-based protein powder
½ cup (45 g) gluten-free quick oats
1 teaspoon chia seeds
½ teaspoon ground cinnamon
½ teaspoon vanilla extract
¼ cup (40 g) fresh berries (or seasonal fruit of choice), plus extra to garnish
1 teaspoon sliced almonds, plus extra to garnish (optional)
1 teaspoon crushed walnuts, plus extra to garnish (optional)

In a blender, blend your coconut milk and protein powder until thoroughly combined. Scoop the mixture into a large bowl, add the other ingredients, and mix well (alternatively, use a large mason jar, screw close, and shake it up). Chill in the refrigerator for 20 minutes while you take a shower in the morning, or for maximum creaminess, leave it overnight and have it for breakfast the following day.

To serve, place into a serving bowl and garnish with extra berries and nuts—it'll make breakfast feel like a treat.

"

I am grounded in possibility.

GET CREATIVE:
Have fun mixing and matching flavors with your protein powder and fruit. I love my chocolate protein with strawberries or raspberries, while I really enjoy vanilla protein with peaches or blueberries! Spice it up by trying different combos till you find something you love.

Meditation for Balancing the Nervous Energies

Sit comfortably. With your elbows out, connect your hands a few inches in front of your heart center, palms facing the chest. Place the palm of your right hand against the back of your left hand. Keep your hands and forearms parallel to the ground so that the fingers of the right hand point toward the left side and the fingers of the left hand point toward the right side. Press your thumb tips together. Close your eyes almost all the way, leaving just a slit of light coming through. Inhale deeply through your nose and hold the breath in for 15 to 20 seconds, then exhale through the nose and hold the breath out for 15 to 20 seconds. Continue for 3 minutes. To close the meditation, take a deep breath in, hold it, exhale, and relax.

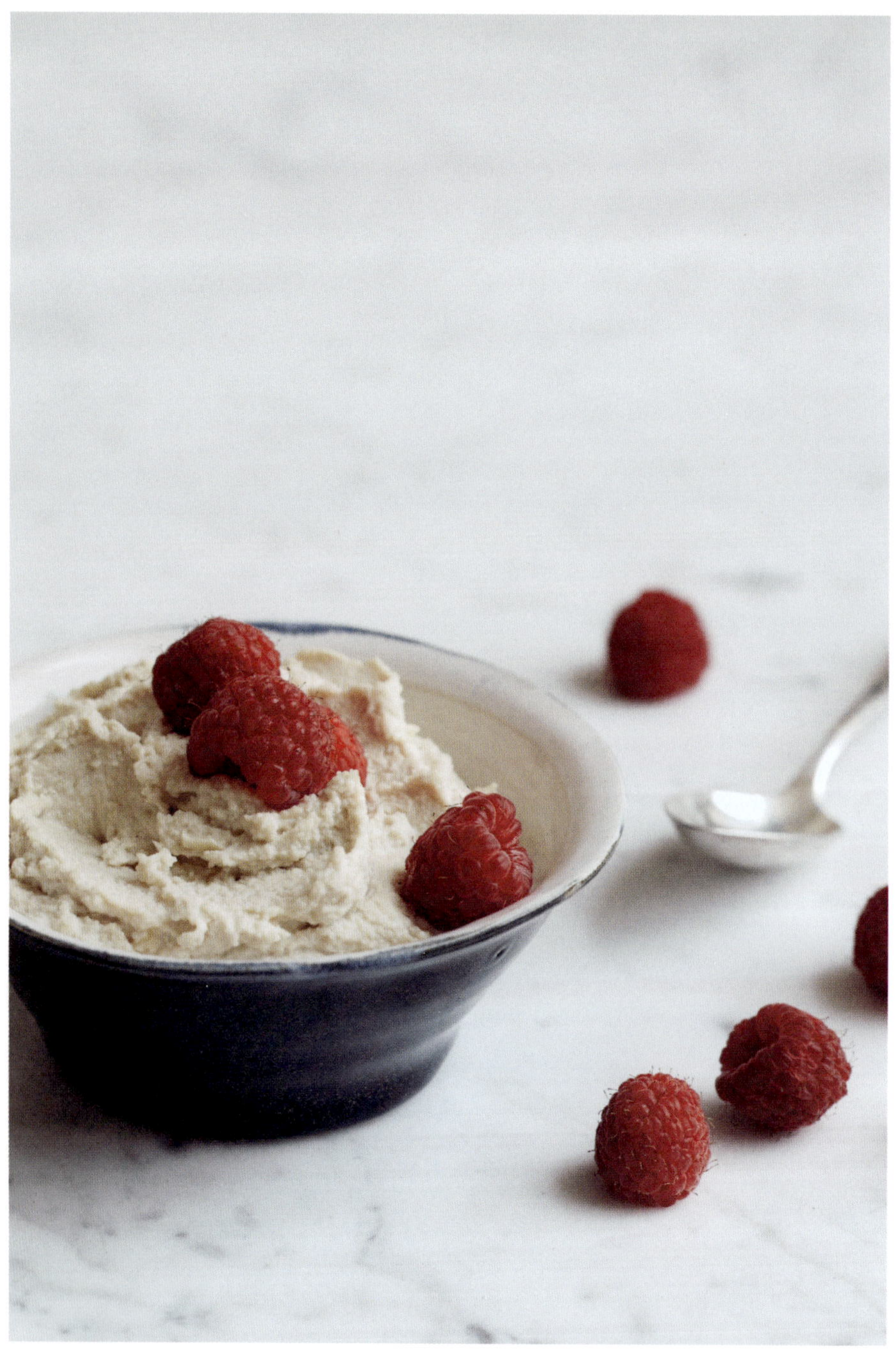

Creamy Cashew Yogurt

Whatever is happening in your life, it's happening for you, not to you. Release your expectations and empower yourself to make the best of what is. When I first started toying around with making an alternative yogurt, I had no idea how it would turn out. But I soon discovered that cashews make a perfect dairy-free Greek "yogurt." Keep a big batch in the fridge and toss some berries and granola in as you move through your week.

YIELD: 6 servings

1½ cups (195 g) raw unsalted cashew nuts
Juice of 1 lemon
1/3 cup (80 ml) canned coconut milk
1 tablespoon (15 ml) vanilla extract
Raspberries, to serve (optional)

In a bowl, combine the cashew nuts and enough cold water to cover and soak for 2 to 3 hours. Drain.

Combine all the ingredients in a food processor or blender and purée until the mixture has a yogurt-like consistency.

Garnish with raspberries, if desired, and serve.

Placing it on the Altar Meditation

Sit in a comfortable position, place your palms facing up on your knees, and start breathing in through your nose and out through your mouth. Focus on your heart center and visualize a golden ball of light that grows with each inhale and exhale until it surrounds your entire being in a bubble.

Now, welcome into your bubble your higher power and any angels, guides, or loved ones you would like to support you. Visualize an altar in front of you and your divine support system all around you. In their loving presence, place the situation you are trying to control on the altar. Feel yourself surrendering this situation to your higher power and releasing your need to figure out how it will come to pass. Open yourself to receive any wisdom or guidance about this situation while you are in this sacred space. When you are ready, thank your divine support team for taking this situation off your hands.

Finally, bring your awareness back to your heart center as you shrink that bubble of golden light back into your being, feeling lighter and more at peace. Repeat this meditation if you find yourself trying to micromanage the situation again.

"

I release my expectations.

Feel-Good Fuel Bars

We need to fill our cup so that it can overflow into the world, because if we are drained and depleted, everyone loses! Nourishing your mind, body, and soul has a tremendous effect on how you interact with everyone you encounter during your day. These feel-good bars are super addictive, delicious, and nourishing, and perfect for a meal on the go.

YIELD: 12 to 15 bars

1 teaspoon flaxseed meal
1 tablespoon (15 ml) water
2 tablespoons (24 g) raw extra-virgin coconut oil, divided
2 cups (192 g) gluten-free oats
¾ cup (67 g) dried goji berries (or your favorite dried fruit)
⅓ cup (80 ml) brown-rice syrup
¼ cup (60 ml) unsweetened almond milk
¼ cup (40 g) hemp protein powder
3 tablespoons (30 g) hemp hearts
2 tablespoons (32 g) cashew butter
3 tablespoons (19 g) halved walnuts
3 tablespoons (13 g) sliced almonds
3 tablespoons (13 g) coconut flakes
3 tablespoons (26 g) chopped raw unsalted cashew nuts
3 tablespoons (12 g) pumpkin seeds
3 tablespoons (25 g) sunflower seeds
4 ounces (112 g) vegan sugar-free chocolate chips

To make the flax "egg," mix together the flaxseed and water in a small bowl and set aside for 5 minutes, until thickened.

Preheat the oven to 425°F (220°C, or gas mark 7). Grease a medium baking pan with 1 tablespoon (12 g) coconut oil.

In a large bowl, combine the flax "egg" and remaining ingredients and mix thoroughly, until it is clumpy and granola-like in texture.

Pour onto the baking pan and spread evenly. Bake in the oven for 5 to 10 minutes, or until the edges begin to toast. (Keep an eye on them and be sure they do not brown.) Set aside to cool.

Use a sharp knife or pizza cutter to cut the granola into 12 to 15 squares.

GET CREATIVE:
Make these bars your own by sticking to the measurements but utilizing your favorite nuts, dried fruit, seeds, protein powder, etc. I love making this recipe to use up the last little bits of ingredients that are cluttering up my pantry. You can also swap some of the nuts for puffed quinoa or buckwheat groats to make a version that's lower in fat if your body is craving something lighter.

"

I am taking care of myself.

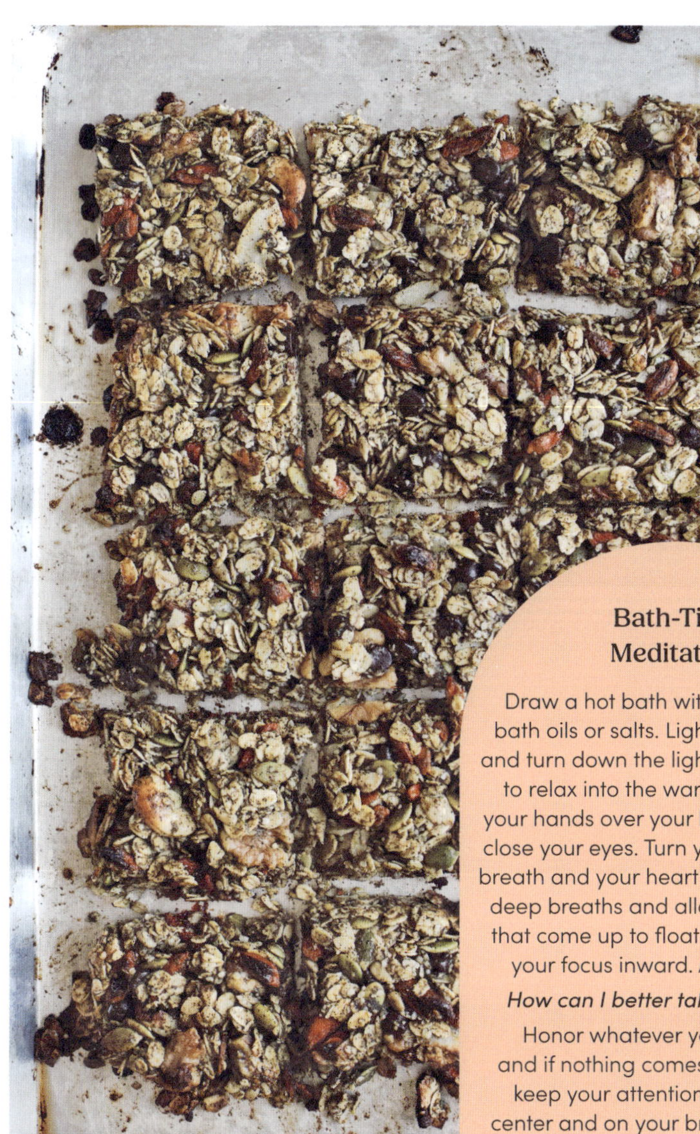

Bath-Time Meditation

Draw a hot bath with your favorite bath oils or salts. Light some candles and turn down the lights. Allow yourself to relax into the warm water, place your hands over your heart center, and close your eyes. Turn your focus to your breath and your heart space. Take long, deep breaths and allow any thoughts that come up to float on by, returning your focus inward. Ask your body,

How can I better take care of you?

Honor whatever you may hear, and if nothing comes up right away, keep your attention at your heart center and on your breath. Relax and enjoy this loving posture. When you are ready to close the meditation, take a deep breath in and hold it, feeling loving energy from your heart center circulate throughout your body, and then release.

Veggie Tom Kha

We may not know how to get around a block, but we know there is always a way through. You can handle this. This soup recipe came about after I found my way through one of my own blocks. Thai cooking really used to intimidate me—but once I got out of my own way and let myself play in the kitchen, magic was made.

YIELD: 4 servings

1 14-ounce package (397 g) extra-firm tofu, drained and cut into 3-inch cubes
¼ cup (59 ml) coconut aminos (or tamari)
1 teaspoon extra-virgin olive oil
3 cups (720 ml) vegetable broth
2 stalks lemongrass, cut into 1-inch sections
1 white onion, thinly sliced
4-inch (10 cm) piece galangal or ginger root, thinly sliced
2 cups (476 ml) canned coconut milk
3 bird's-eye chiles, halved
Juice of 1 lime
1 cup (70 g) chopped cremini mushrooms
3 tablespoons (45 ml) tamari (gluten-free soy sauce)
3 tablespoons (3 g) chopped cilantro, plus extra to garnish
1 bag shiritaki or rice noodles (optional)

Toss the tofu with the coconut aminos and olive oil. You can bake the tofu cubes at 350°F (180°C, or gas mark 4) for 10 minutes or place in an air fryer for 5 minutes at 450°F (232°C).

While the tofu is baking, combine the vegetable broth, lemongrass, onion, and galangal in a large saucepan and bring to a boil over medium heat. Reduce the heat and simmer for 2 to 3 minutes, stirring continuously. Add the coconut milk, chiles, lime juice, mushrooms, tamari, and cilantro and continue to simmer for another 5 to 7 minutes. Add shiritaki or rice noodles, if using.

Ladle into individual bowls, garnish with cilantro, and serve hot. If you don't want the soup to be fiery hot, remove the chiles before serving.

Inner Conflict Resolver Meditation

Set the intention for your meditation before beginning. What would you like guidance on? Surrender it as you move into the meditation.

Sit comfortably, with your eyes almost closed. Place your hands over your chest, palms on your torso and fingers pointing toward each other across the chest. Turn your attention to the breath. Inhale deeply for 5 seconds. Exhale completely for 5 seconds. Hold the breath out for 15 seconds as you pull in your navel point and abdomen. Begin with 11 minutes, gradually building up to 31 or 62 minutes if you feel called. To close, take a deep inhale and stretch your arms up over your head. Return to breathing naturally and shake your arms and hands for 15 to 30 seconds. Relax.

"

I sit in the knowing that there is a way through every block.

Watermelon Gazpacho

Decide that you are ready for change and open yourself up to moving through it with love, grace, and ease. This soup inspired the topic of change because I was not into gazpachos, but when I put my own remix on it, I ended up falling head over heels for this "out-of-my-comfort-zone" soup. I hope you do, too!

YIELD: 4 servings

2 cups (304 g) chopped watermelon
2 red bell peppers, seeded and roughly chopped
1 green apple, peeled and roughly chopped, divided
1 cucumber, peeled and roughly chopped, divided
½ white onion, diced
¼ cup (60 ml) extra-virgin olive oil
2 tablespoons (30 ml) balsamic vinegar
2 tablespoons (8 g) finely chopped fresh mint, divided

In a blender or food processor, combine the watermelon, bell peppers, half the apple, half the cucumber, and onion. Add the olive oil, balsamic vinegar, and 1 tablespoon (4 g) chopped mint. Purée until thick and smooth.

Pour the gazpacho into serving bowls. Stir in the remaining apple and cucumber. Sprinkle over the remaining 1 tablespoon (4 g) mint. Chill before serving!

Kundalini Meditation for Change

Sit in a comfortable position with your chest lifted. With your eyes closed, start long, deep breathing, and follow the flow of your breath. Curl your fingers in as if making a fist, then bring your hands together at the center of your chest. The hands should touch lightly in two places only: the knuckles of the middle fingers and the pads of the thumbs. Your thumbs are extended toward your heart center and are pressed together. Hold this position and feel the energy across the thumbs and knuckles. It is recommended to do this meditation for 31 minutes; however, if you are just starting out, try the meditation for 5 or 11 minutes, gradually building up to a full 31-minute practice if you desire. To close, inhale deeply, exhale, and relax for 5 minutes.

"

I am ready for change.

Asian Broccoli Slaw

This delicious dish can help you create momentum in the kitchen. Not only is it nourishing and satisfying, but it's also creative enough to get your culinary juices flowing. It's paired with a meditation for busting through blocks, creating momentum, and freeing us from the subconscious thought patterns and habits that we are addicted to but that aren't serving us. It's the first meditation I do each morning to ease into my practice.

YIELD: 1 serving (per option)

12-ounce (340 g) bag broccoli slaw
¼ cup (50 g) shelled edamame
¼ cup (10 g) shredded radicchio
¼ cup (18 g) slivered almonds, plus extra to garnish
¼ cup (27 g) shredded carrot, plus extra to garnish
½ cup (93 g) cooked quinoa

DRESSING

¼ cup (60 ml) macadamia nut oil (or extra-virgin olive oil)
3 tablespoons (45 ml) rice vinegar
3 tablespoons (45 ml) sesame oil
3 tablespoons (45 ml) shoyu (or soy sauce)
3 cloves garlic, finely chopped
1 tablespoon (6 g) chopped scallion
1 tablespoon (6 g) grated fresh ginger

To make the dressing, combine all the dressing ingredients and whisk until well blended.

Put the broccoli slaw, edamame, radicchio, almonds, and carrots in a large bowl and toss to mix.

Drizzle enough dressing into the slaw mixture so that the slaw is damp but not soaked.

Put the quinoa on a plate and top with the broccoli slaw mixture.

Garnish with extra almond slivers and shredded carrots, if desired.

Kundalini Meditation for Addictions

Sit comfortably with your eyes closed and focus on your third-eye point. Make fists with both of your hands and extend the thumbs out straight. Place your thumbs on your temples and find the niches where your thumbs fit in. Lock your upper and lower molars together and keep your lips closed. Keeping your teeth pressed together throughout, alternately squeeze the molars tightly and then release the pressure. Muscles will move in rhythm under your thumbs. Feel them massage the thumbs and apply pressure to the temples with your hands. Silently vibrate the four primal sounds:

sa ta na ma

Continue for 3 minutes, then take a deep breath in and hold it. Exhale and bring your hands down.

"

I create momentum through action.

California Kale Salad

Honoring my inner voice has my number one secret to creating a life that lights me up, and my inner voice encouraged me to move to California. This recipe is your quintessential kale salad with my personal spin on it—a combination of all my favorite things: creamy avocado, crunchy nuts, sweet berries, satiating tempeh, and light and tangy homemade vinaigrette.

YIELD: 2 servings

8 ounces (227 g) tempeh, cut into 3-inch cubes
1 tablespoon (15 ml) extra-virgin olive oil
¼ cup coconut aminos
½ teaspoon garlic powder
½ teaspoon onion powder
½ teaspoon paprika
2 cups (136 g) chopped baby kale
3 tablespoons (13 g) sliced almonds, plus extra to garnish
2 tablespoons (20 g) hemp hearts
1 avocado, halved, pitted, and sliced
½ cup (83 g) chopped strawberries

DRESSING
2 heaping tablespoons (30 g) tahini
2 heaping tablespoons (30 g) Dijon mustard
¼ cup (60 ml) extra-virgin olive oil
¼ cup (60 ml) balsamic vinegar

To make the dressing, combine all ingredients in a small bowl and whisk together until creamy. Set aside.

Add the tempeh to a small bowl with the olive oil, coconut aminos, and spices and mix to coat the tempeh. Sauté the tempeh in a small saucepan over medium-low heat by moving it around with a spatula until it starts to brown. (You can also air-fry it for 5 minutes at 450°F or 232°C.)

In a large bowl, combine the tempeh and the remaining ingredients, drizzle over the dressing, and toss until the salad is thoroughly dressed. Transfer to a serving bowl and garnish with the nuts.

Intuitive Meditation and Writing

Grab a pen and paper and find a comfortable spot. Write down a question about something in your life that you've been struggling with. Now close your eyes, place your palms face up, and bring your attention to your natural breathing. Imagine a ray of light coming down from the sky, into the top of your head, or crown chakra, and pouring its beam of light into your heart center. With each breath, see this light filling you up with its energy. Continue for 3 minutes. At the end of the 3 minutes, take a deep breath in and hold it, feeling the light saturate every particle of your being, then exhale. Now immediately put your pen to paper and answer your question. Don't think; just allow whatever is coming forth flow outward. Keep writing until you feel complete and then go back and look at the guidance you have received on the matter.

"

I honor my inner voice.

Brussels Sprout Tacos

When I think about being in love with the little things in life, brussels sprouts, avocados, and tacos come to my mind.

YIELD: 4 tacos

½ cup (44 g) chopped brussels sprouts
1 tablespoon (15 g) Dijon mustard or horseradish
½ teaspoon garlic powder
½ teaspoon onion powder
Salt and freshly ground black pepper, to taste
Coconut oil cooking spray, for greasing
4 to 6 slices (¼ inch, or 6 mm, thick) tempeh or extra-firm tofu, cut into bite-sized pieces
3 tablespoons (45 ml) organic barbecue sauce or garlic teriyaki sauce
4 flour tortillas (or corn for gluten-free)
2 romaine lettuce leaves, shredded
1 medium carrot, shredded
1 avocado, halved, pitted, and sliced
1 shallot, thinly sliced

In a medium bowl, combine the brussels sprouts, Dijon or horseradish, garlic powder, onion powder, and a little salt and pepper and mix well until the brussels sprouts are thoroughly coated.

Spray a little cooking spray on a medium frying pan and gently sauté the brussels sprouts for 5 to 7 minutes, or until lightly browned. Set aside.

Heat the tempeh or tofu in a nonstick frying pan over medium heat and add the barbecue or garlic teriyaki sauce. Stir for 5 minutes, or until heated through and slightly crisp.

Place a tortilla in a dry frying pan over medium heat and cook for about 45 seconds on each side, until warm and lightly brown. Repeat with the remaining tortillas.

Place the lettuce in the center of a tortilla, and then add the carrots, brussels sprouts, and tempeh or tofu. Top with slices of avocado and shallots, and then wrap closed.

“

I am in love with the little things.

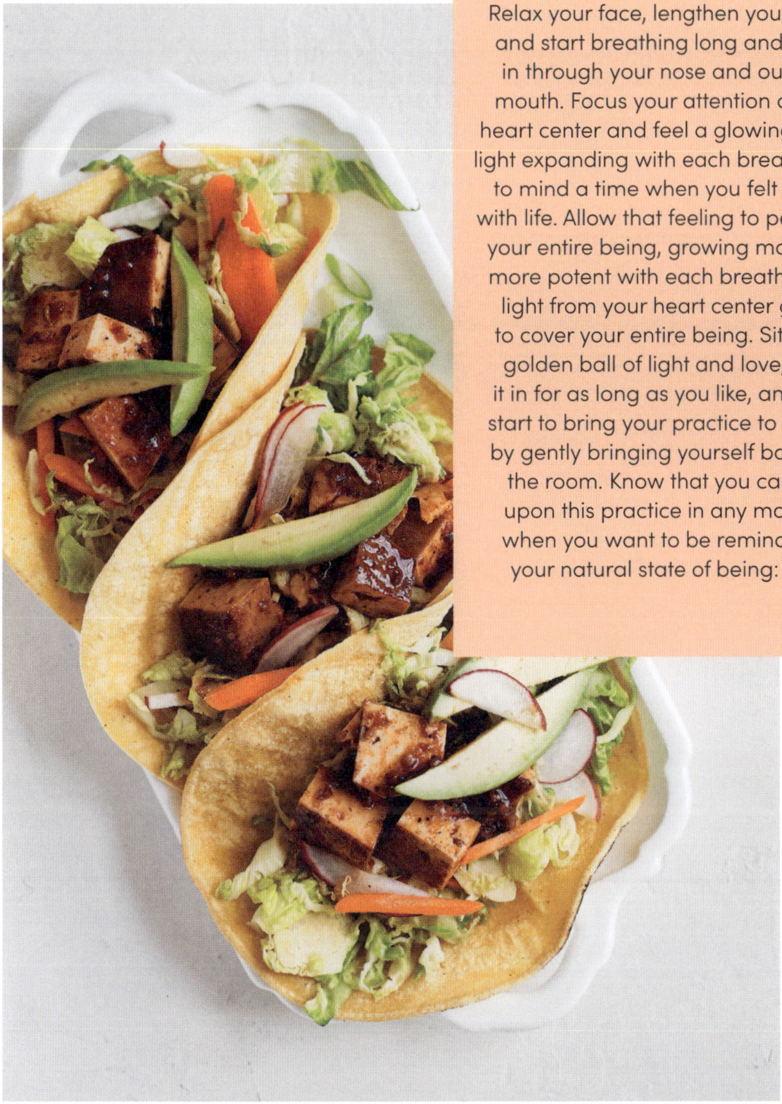

Loving the Moment Meditation

Sit comfortably and close your eyes. Relax your face, lengthen your spine, and start breathing long and deep, in through your nose and out your mouth. Focus your attention at your heart center and feel a glowing ball of light expanding with each breath. Bring to mind a time when you felt in love with life. Allow that feeling to permeate your entire being, growing more and more potent with each breath as the light from your heart center grows to cover your entire being. Sit in this golden ball of light and love, soak it in for as long as you like, and then start to bring your practice to a close by gently bringing yourself back into the room. Know that you can call upon this practice in any moment when you want to be reminded of your natural state of being: love.

Mexican Quinoa Avocado Boats

What are you truly desiring when you start to feel hungry? What could you incorporate into your life that would provide real nourishment? These fun avocado boats will leave you feeling satisfied and nourished! The accompanying meditation (on the following page) will help you feed your soul as well as your body.

YIELD: 8 boats

½ cup (85 g) uncooked quinoa, soaked in water
Pinch of salt
1 cup (240 ml) water
½ cup (97 g) precooked black beans, soaked in water
½ cup precooked corn
½ yellow pepper, chopped
½ red pepper, chopped
½ red onion, diced
¼ cup (4 g) chopped cilantro
¼ cup (60 ml) chile-infused macadamia nut oil or extra-virgin olive oil
Juice of ½ lime
4 ripe avocados

Drain the quinoa, and then place it in a medium saucepan along with a pinch of salt and the water. Bring to a boil, reduce the heat, and simmer for about 15 minutes, until cooked through and fluffy.

Meanwhile, drain the black beans and place them into a medium mixing bowl. Add the corn, chopped peppers, red onion, and cilantro.

Add the cooked quinoa, oil, and lime juice to the mixing bowl and stir. Cut the avocados in half, remove the seed, and scoop in the quinoa mixture. Voilà—simple, fun, and totally adorable healthy meal.

NOTE:
If you're bringing these to a barbecue or leaving them out at a dinner, drizzle extra lime juice over the avocado to prevent it from browning.

"

I am nourished by my passion.

Meditation for Soul Nourishment

Find a comfortable spot in your home and lay a few special things in front of you. I recommend a candle, a picture of someone who inspires you (or an angel, guru, or guide of your preference), a few precious trinkets. Doing this helps you create a special moment for yourself and allows you to tune into your intuition. Have a notebook or a few sheets of paper on hand for afterward, in case you want to write what has come up for you.

Sit in a comfortable seated position with your palms facing up on your knees and your spine held straight and elongated. Take a deep breath. Feel your body relax and your heart space expand with each new breath. Notice the innate sense of love and support you have inside. Allow yourself to sit in it for a little while. When you are ready, ask from deep within for whatever nourishment you need. Ask where in your life you can infuse more passion—where have you been neglecting your passions? Allow yourself to inquire for a moment or two, and then sit back in the silence. Return your focus to your heart center and just breathe, listening for what comes up for the next 3 to 5 minutes. To close the meditation, take a deep breath in with gratitude for the wisdom shared, and exhale. Relax, then jot down any revelations in your notebook. If nothing comes up for you, don't worry; you have raised the question, so simply stay open for the day ahead and let yourself receive the guidance brought to you throughout the day!

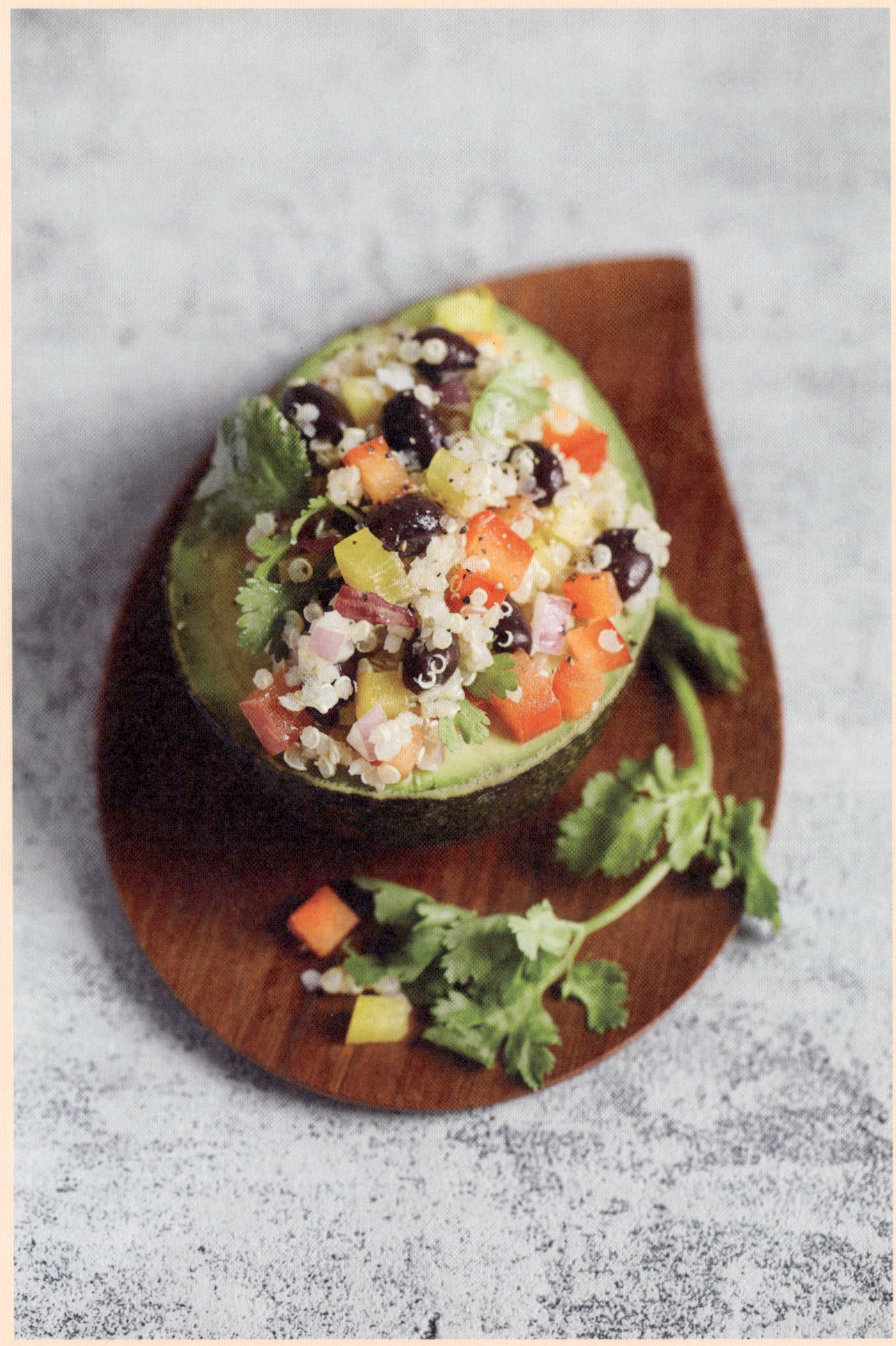

Veggie Burger and Avocado Fries

Our perfectionism paralyzes us. Case in point: I had to step away from this recipe for a while because I was stressing over getting it right. When I did come back to it, I released all expectations, picked a completely different set of ingredients, and let myself have fun. It turned out to be the best thing I've ever tasted!

YIELD: 12 burgers

BURGERS
1 tablespoon (9 g) flaxseed meal
3 tablespoons (45 ml) water
Olive oil cooking spray, for greasing
1 bulb garlic, cloves separated and peeled
1 cup (164 g) precooked chickpeas
½ cup (35 g) cremini mushrooms
⅓ cup (80 g) Dijon mustard
1 tablespoon (15 ml) extra-virgin olive oil
2 teaspoons dried oregano
1 teaspoon ground turmeric
1 teaspoon onion powder
1 teaspoon salt
½ teaspoon black pepper
1 cup (200 g) cooked green lentils
1 cup (186 g) cooked quinoa (or "super-grain" blend of quinoa, millet, and buckwheat)
½ cup (56 g) quinoa flour
12 gluten-free rolls, to serve
Baby kale, to serve
Sliced red onions, to serve

SAUCE
3 tablespoons (45 g) eggless mayonnaise
1 tablespoon (16 g) tomato paste
1 teaspoon grated fresh horseradish

AVOCADO FRIES
Coconut oil, for greasing
2 tablespoons (30 ml) extra-virgin olive oil
2 tablespoons (18 g) flaxseed meal
6 tablespoons (90 ml) water
1 cup (60 g) panko bread crumbs
1 teaspoon onion powder
1 teaspoon salt, plus extra to taste
Freshly ground black pepper, to taste
1 teaspoon garlic powder
2 near-ripe avocados, halved and pitted

"

I release the need to be perfect.

To make the flax "egg," mix together the flaxseed and water in a small bowl and set aside for 5 minutes, until thickened.

To make the burgers, preheat the oven to 375°F (190°C, or gas mark 5). Lightly grease a baking sheet with the cooking spray. Set aside.

Wrap the peeled garlic cloves in a small piece of foil, and place them in the oven for 20 minutes to roast.

In a food processor, combine the flax "egg," chickpeas, mushrooms, mustard, olive oil, spices, and roasted garlic, and pulse together until thoroughly combined. Transfer the mixture to a medium mixing bowl and add the lentils and quinoa. Using a spoon or your hands, thoroughly combine the mixture and gradually add the quinoa flour, a little at a time, until the mixture is thickened but still moist.

Shape a heaping spoonful of the mixture into a ball, just slightly bigger than a golf ball. Place it onto the prepared baking sheet and flatten it out into a patty. Repeat with the remaining mixture (you should have about a dozen burgers—I always freeze at least half and keep some in the fridge for later in the week). Bake for 20 minutes, or until the outer edges lose their moisture and appear on the drier side.

To make the sauce, combine all the ingredients together and mix well.

Separate a gluten-free bun and place it on a plate. Put a patty on one side, top with a generous slathering of sauce, baby kale, and red onion slices.

To make the fries, preheat the oven to 425°F (220°C, or gas mark 7). Lightly grease a baking sheet with coconut oil.

In one bowl, whisk together the flaxseed meal and water. In another bowl, mix your panko and seasonings. Slice the avocados lengthwise, dip them in the flaxseed mixture, and then into the panko mixture.

Place on the prepared baking sheet and adjust the seasoning to taste. I like to add a couple more shakes of garlic and onion powder and a little more salt before they go in the oven. Bake for 10 minutes, or until the panko starts to brown. Any extra sauce can be used for dipping!

Bath-Time Reflection

Take a bath or a shower this evening with the intention of reflecting on what you would do differently if you didn't care about being perfect. What would you reach for or express if you were okay with showing up in the messy middle? Where do you hold yourself back because you don't feel like you have it all figured out yet?

Let yourself relax and honor whatever thoughts, feelings and images naturally arise in your mind and body. When you've received some insight, allow yourself to feel the water cleansing you of the perfectionism that's blocking you. Surrender all the fears that come up around moving towards your desires and emerge free and clean to move forward.

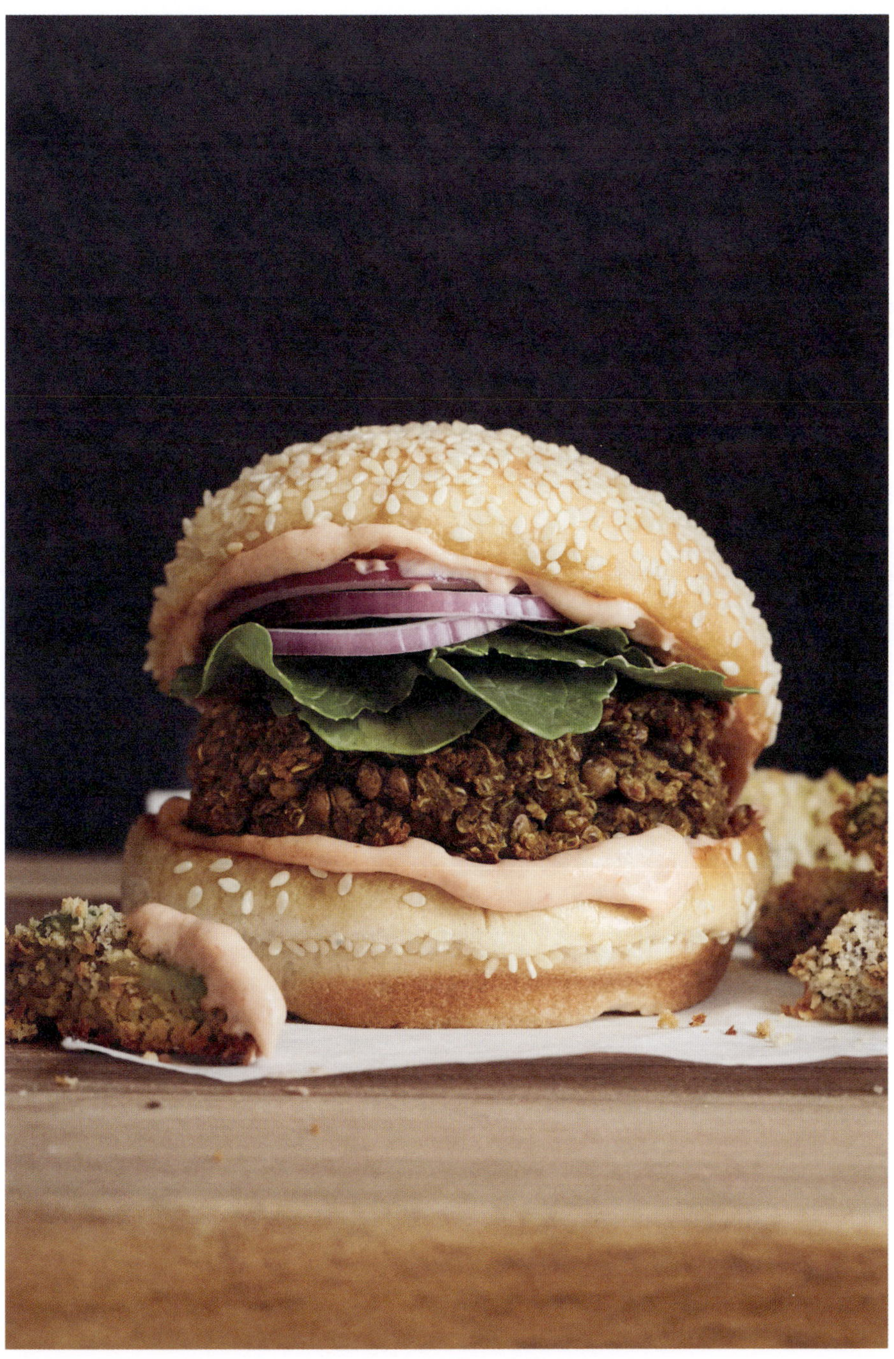

Key Lime Pie Bars

We may think we want the sweet parts of our lives all the time—the happiness, excitement, and success—but it's the sour that helps us appreciate the sweet. And key lime pie is the perfect combination of sour and sweet to help us appreciate both!

YIELD: 12 bars

CRUST
1¼ cups (124 g) whole pecans
2 tablespoons (32 g) cashew butter
1 cup (175 g) pitted dates
1 tablespoon (12 g) raw extra-virgin coconut oil, for greasing

FILLING
1 ripe avocado, halved, pitted, and sliced
1½ cups (195 g) raw unsalted cashew nuts, soaked in water for 2 to 3 hours and then drained
⅓ cup (155 ml) key lime juice (about 6 key limes; you can substitute with 6 regular limes and 3 tablespoons, or 45 ml, cassava sweetener added to the juice, or omit it if you prefer a tart pie)

GARNISH
Zest of 2 key limes
12 pecans

To make the crust, combine the pecans, cashew butter, and dates in a food processor and pulse until thoroughly combined and clumpy. Grease a 12-cup muffin tray with coconut oil and then lay down the crust mix inside each cup, until 1 inch (2.5 cm) deep. Place the tray, flat, in the freezer while preparing the filling.

Clean the food processor, then add the avocado, cashews, and lime juice to the processor and pulse until a nice creamy mixture is created.

Remove the pan from the freezer and scoop about 2 tablespoons (30 g) filling into each cup. Garnish with the lime zest and a pecan and serve.

"

I appreciate both the sweet and sour in my life.

Meditation for Holding Both Sides

Sit cross-legged. Place your palms facing up on each knee. Start deepening your breath and turn your attention inwards, assessing. Now bring your attention to your palms. In your right hand, feel yourself holding all the "sour" things in your life—the challenges, frustrations, or things you wish were different. Don't judge them or try to change them, just let them be held in your right palm. Next, bring awareness to your left palm, allowing your "sweet" things to be held here—the joys, the wins, the things you are grateful for. Now, take the next 5 to 10 minutes to hold both simultaneously. Observe how the two balance each other, how the sour gives perspective on the sweet. Notice what arises from holding both sides. To close, bring both hands together at your heart center and take a deep inhale, hold it for 15 seconds, and exhale to release.

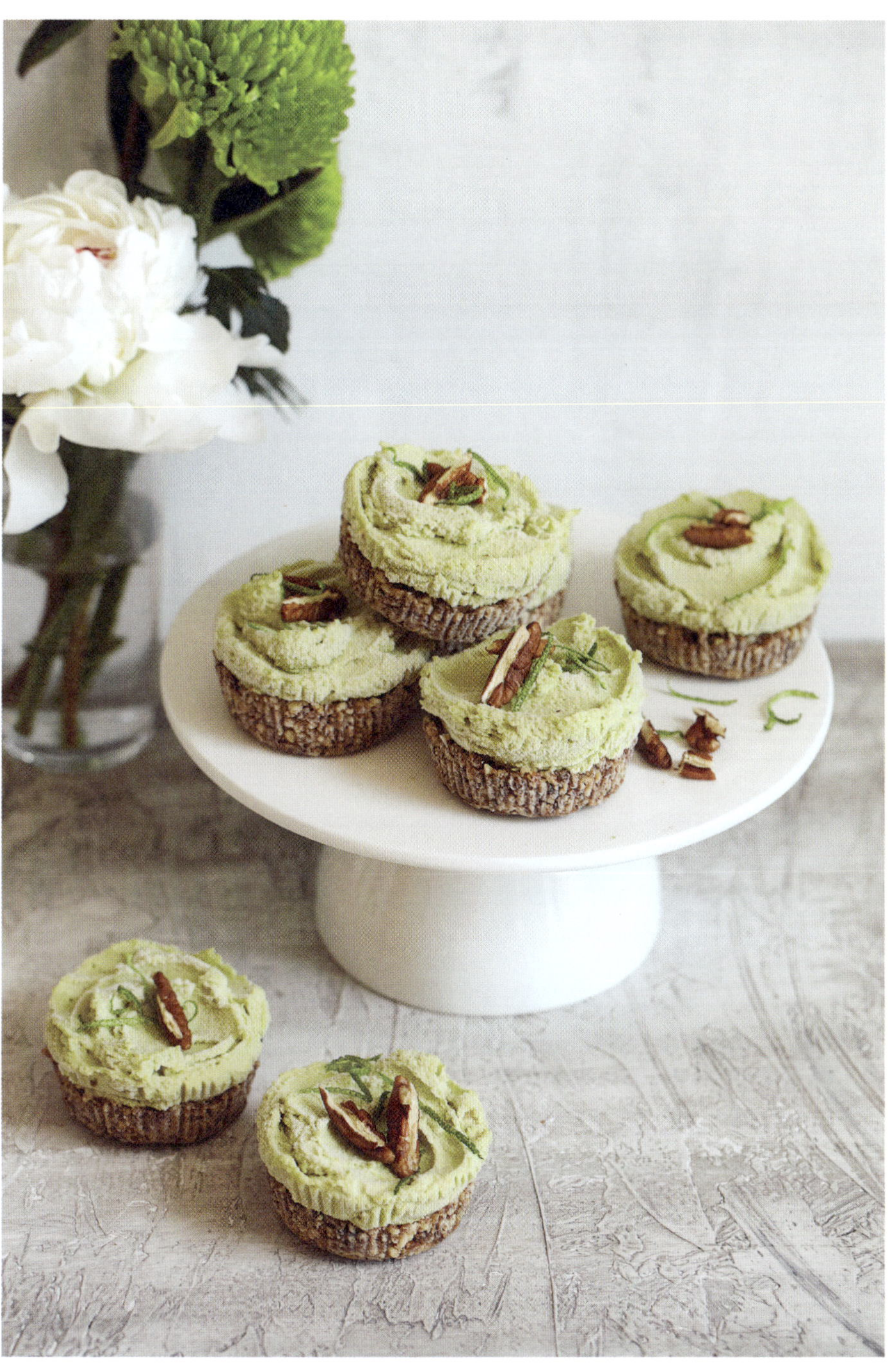

Mixed Berry Tartlets

There is nothing more attractive than being unapologetically you. Your authenticity makes you magnetic! I love how this tart is simply highlighting the natural, multifaceted flavors of the berries. The crust alone is spiced, so the sweetness of the fruit in the filling really stands out.

YIELD: 12 tartlets

CRUST

1 tablespoon (14 g) vegan butter, melted, for greasing
1½ cups (222 g) gluten-free 1-to-1 flour
3 tablespoons (29 g) date sugar (coconut or maple sugar also work)
1 tablespoon (15 ml) ground cinnamon
½ teaspoon ground nutmeg
1 teaspoon almond extract
¼ cup (56 g) soy-free vegan butter, chilled
3 tablespoons (36 g) raw extra-virgin coconut oil
1 tablespoon (15 ml) apple cider vinegar
¼ cup (60 ml) cold water

FILLING

1 cup (166 g) fresh or frozen strawberries, chopped
1 cup (150 g) fresh or frozen blueberries
1 cup (144 g) fresh or frozen raspberries or blackberries
1 tablespoon (15 ml) vanilla extract
Maple syrup (optional)

GARNISH

¼ cup (25 g) crushed walnuts
¼ cup (18 g) almond slivers
¼ cup (22 g) unsweetened coconut flakes

Preheat the oven to 375°F (190°C, or gas mark 5) and lightly grease a 12-cup muffin pan.

To make the crust, combine all the ingredients in a food processor and pulse until a dough is formed. Roll a small amount of the mixture into a 2-inch (5 cm) ball and spread it out to line the muffin cup. Use a fork to lightly press into the pastry. Repeat with the rest of the dough, and then bake for 15 minutes or until golden.

Meanwhile, make the filling: Combine the berries in a small bowl and add vanilla extract and maple syrup to sweeten, if desired. Scoop a few tablespoons into each cup and bake for another 10 to 15 minutes, or until the edges start to brown.

Garnish with the walnuts, almonds, and coconut flakes!

“

My authenticity is attractive.

Meditation for Authentic Self-Expression

Sit comfortably and place your hands at your heart center, right over left. Close your eyes and sense the area under your palms. Take a steady, powerful breath through the mouth, inhaling first into your chest and then taking a second inhale to fill your belly before letting out a powerful exhale. Hold the intention to witness your most authentic self-expression as you continue this cycle of powerful breath, relaxing and opening to your intuition with each inhale. Continue this pattern of breath for 5 to 10 minutes and then return to your normal breathing.

Let your hands float down to your knees, palms facing up, and bring your awareness to your third eye as you allow yourself to imagine showing up as your most authentic self. Surrender to whatever arises. Stay here for another 5 to 10 minutes. Close by reflecting on what you can do right now to start showing up more authentically in your day-to-day life.

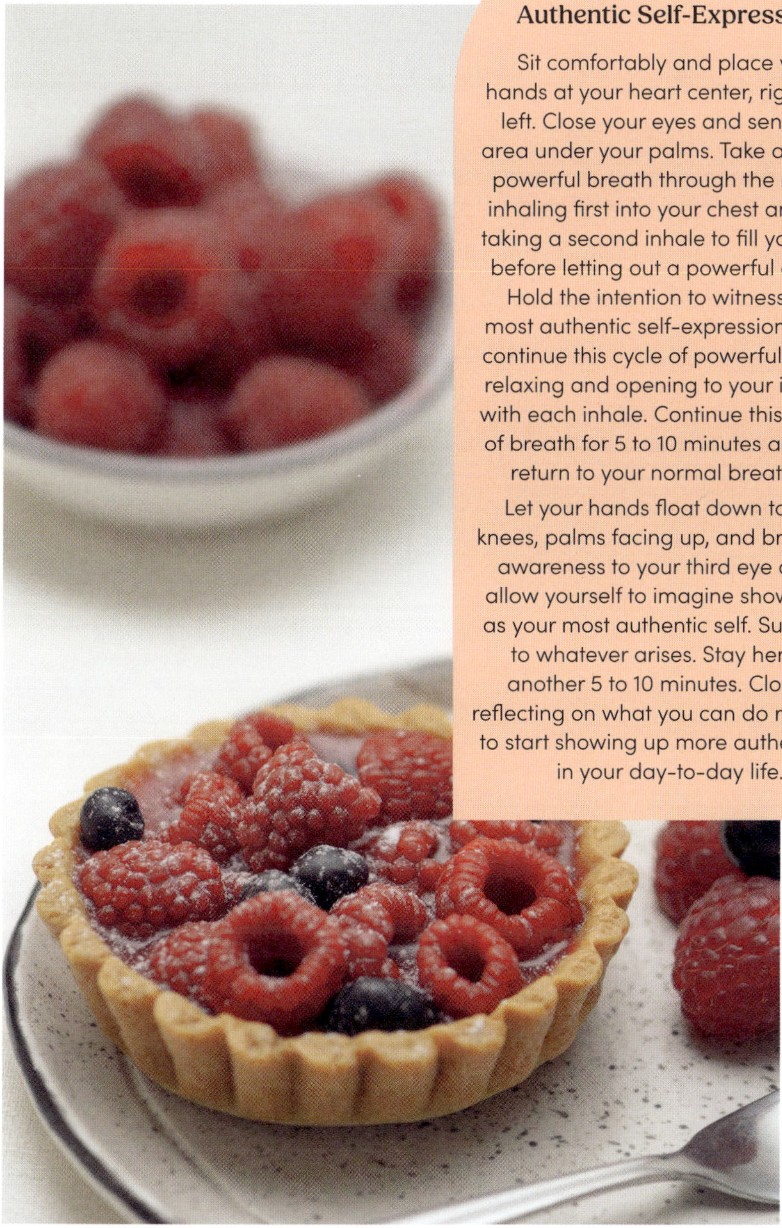

03

Fall

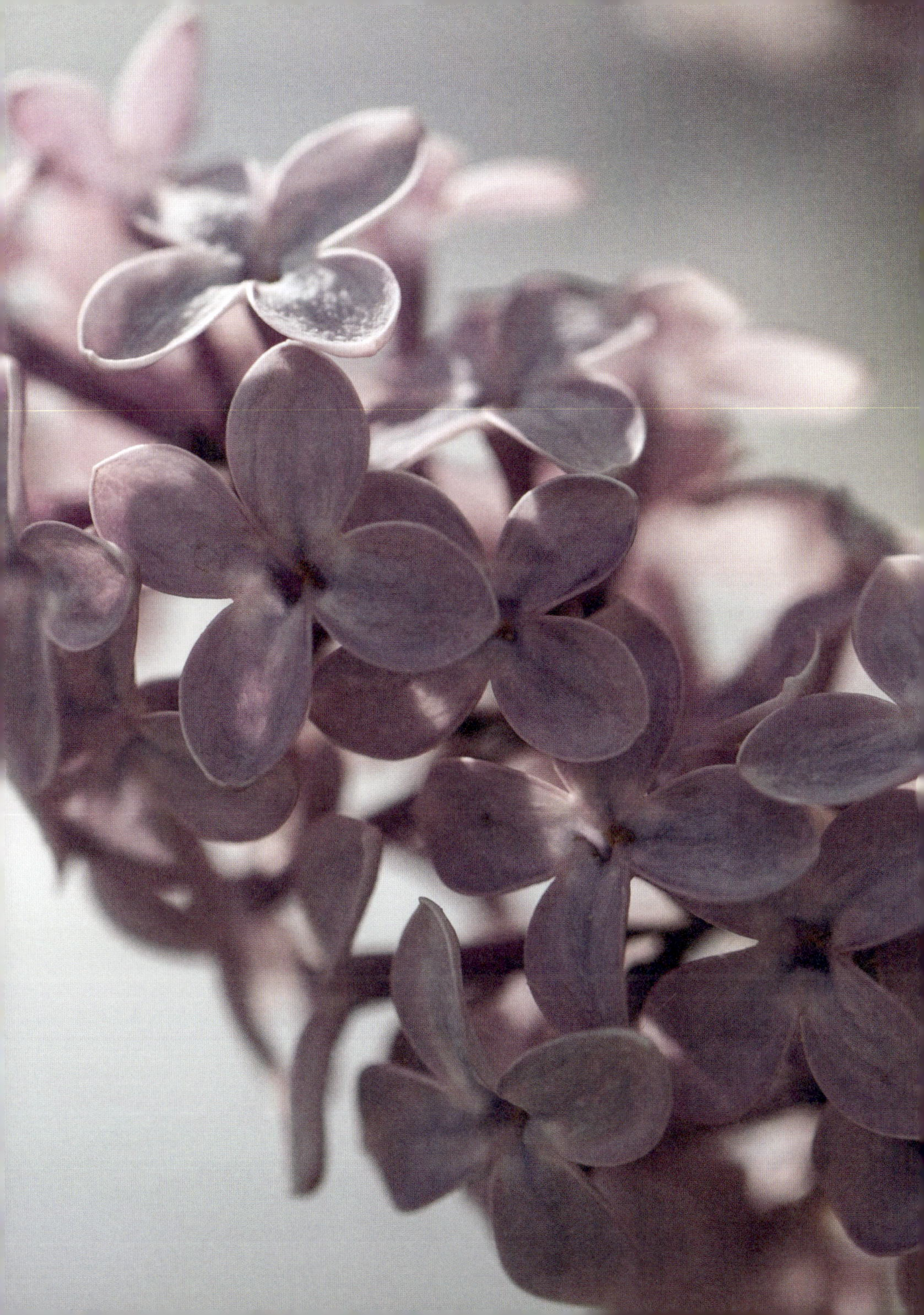

Earthy Juice

Discipline can be your greatest superpower when it comes from a place of self-love. This juice will connect you back to the rooted energy of the Earth. The rich beet and carrots will increase your connection with your natural strength and discipline while the parsley and lemon will detoxify anything in your system that might be getting in your way. Use the paired tapping meditation to touch base with your inner guidance system and offer your mind and body support as you work towards your goals and desires.

YIELD: 1 serving

3 sprigs parsley
2 carrots
1 beet, peeled
1 red apple, coarsely chopped
1 lemon, peeled

Starting with the parsley, juice all the ingredients into a large glass.

Lightly stir and serve immediately.

"

My discipline is rooted in deep self-love.

Tapping Meditation for Discipline

Bring your left hand up to your heart center in a karate chop position with your thumb towards your chest. Begin to tap on the outer side of your left hand, just below your pinky, using the finger pads of your right hand. (You can watch a video demonstration of tapping on my YouTube channel if you are struggling to picture it.) Continue tapping on the side of your left hand while you repeat the below:

I am willing to be disciplined in the pursuit of my highest good and desires, and I love and accept myself.

I am willing to be disciplined in the pursuit of my highest good and desires, and I love and honor myself.

I am willing to be disciplined in the pursuit of my highest good and desires, and I love and forgive myself.

Now, keep tapping as you start speaking aloud about the areas of your life in which you are ready to be more disciplined as well as any reasons you may have struggled to take action in the past. When you feel ready, end your session with:

I release any blocks to discipline for my highest good and desires.

I release all of these blocks from my mind, body, and soul.

I move forward confidently towards my highest good and desires with whatever discipline is needed. And so it is.

Take a deep breath and shake out your hands.

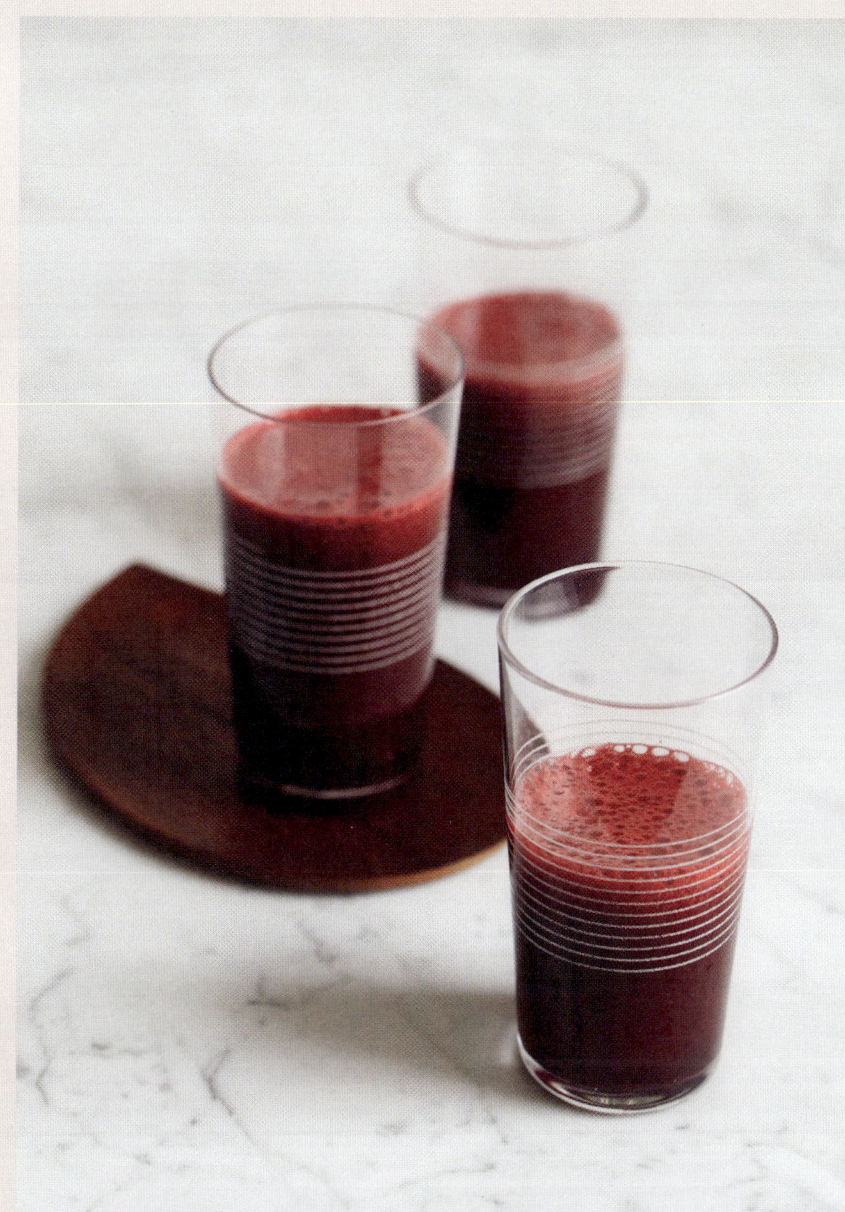

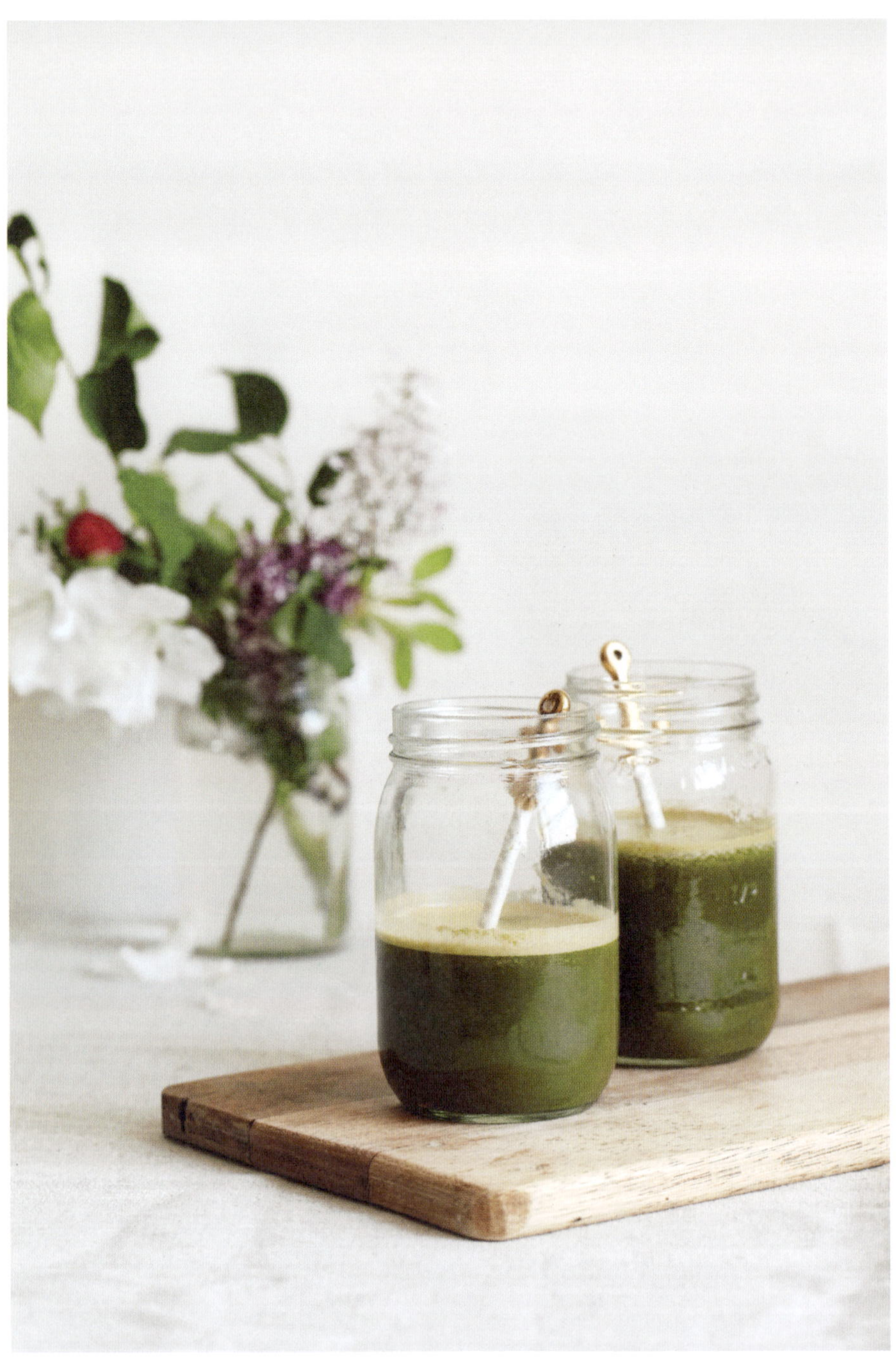

Farmers Market Juice

When you are feeling drained, let nature nourish and recharge you. This juice is packed with a variety of nutrients from some of my go-to veggies, along with ginger and parsley. Experiment with the ingredients that are seasonally available at your local farmers market and make it your own!

YIELD: 1 serving

½ cup (30 g) parsley
8 romaine lettuce leaves
4 carrots
2 apples, coarsely chopped
2 cups (60 g) spinach
1-inch (2.5 cm) piece ginger root

Starting with the parsley, juice all the ingredients into a large glass.

Lightly stir and serve immediately.

Walk in Nature Meditation

Okay, I'm making you get outside for this one! Go to a local garden, park, beach, or even just a path with a lot of trees nearby. If you feel comfortable, take off your shoes and walk barefoot; if not, just imagine that your feet are connected with the ground with each step you take. Turn off your cell phone and put it away. Spend anywhere from 5 to 20 minutes focusing on your breath and taking in the beauty around you. You can also add a silent mantra if you'd like: Simply say to yourself sat on the inhale and nam on the exhale with every step you take. This is a Kundalini mantra that means true self—personally, it grounds me and brings me back to the truth of who I am when I meditate on it.

"

I allow nature to nourish me.

Sunshine Juice

When we choose love, everything feels a whole lot lighter! I originally created this juice to dis-guise the taste of carrot juice, which I don't like. To my surprise, it ended up tasting so good and being such a natural pick-me-up that I nicknamed it my "sunshine juice." I feel like I'm beaming rays of sunshine after I drink it.

YIELD: 1 serving

5 carrots
3 oranges, peeled and quartered
1 grapefruit, peeled and quartered
1 apple, coarsely chopped
1 lemon, peeled

Juice all the ingredients into a large glass. Lightly stir and serve immediately.

Choosing Love Meditation

Sit comfortably. Close your eyes and place your hands at your heart center, right on top of left. Take long, deep breaths in through your nose and out your mouth, feeling the energy in your heart center expand with each breath. Allow any thoughts that have been weighing on you or situations you have been struggling with to float into your mind, one at a time. After seeing the thought, mentally say to yourself,

I could choose love instead of this

Sometimes, the loving solution may pop into your head just as you silently make the declaration; other times, it may be less apparent. Regardless, continue through your grievance inventory for 3 to 5 minutes, mentally saying

I could choose love instead of this

after each thought. When your time is up or you have made it through your list and feel at peace, take a deep breath in, hold it, and say silently,

I let love be my default setting

Allow this belief to saturate your being for the next 10 to 15 seconds. Exhale.

"

I let love be my default setting.

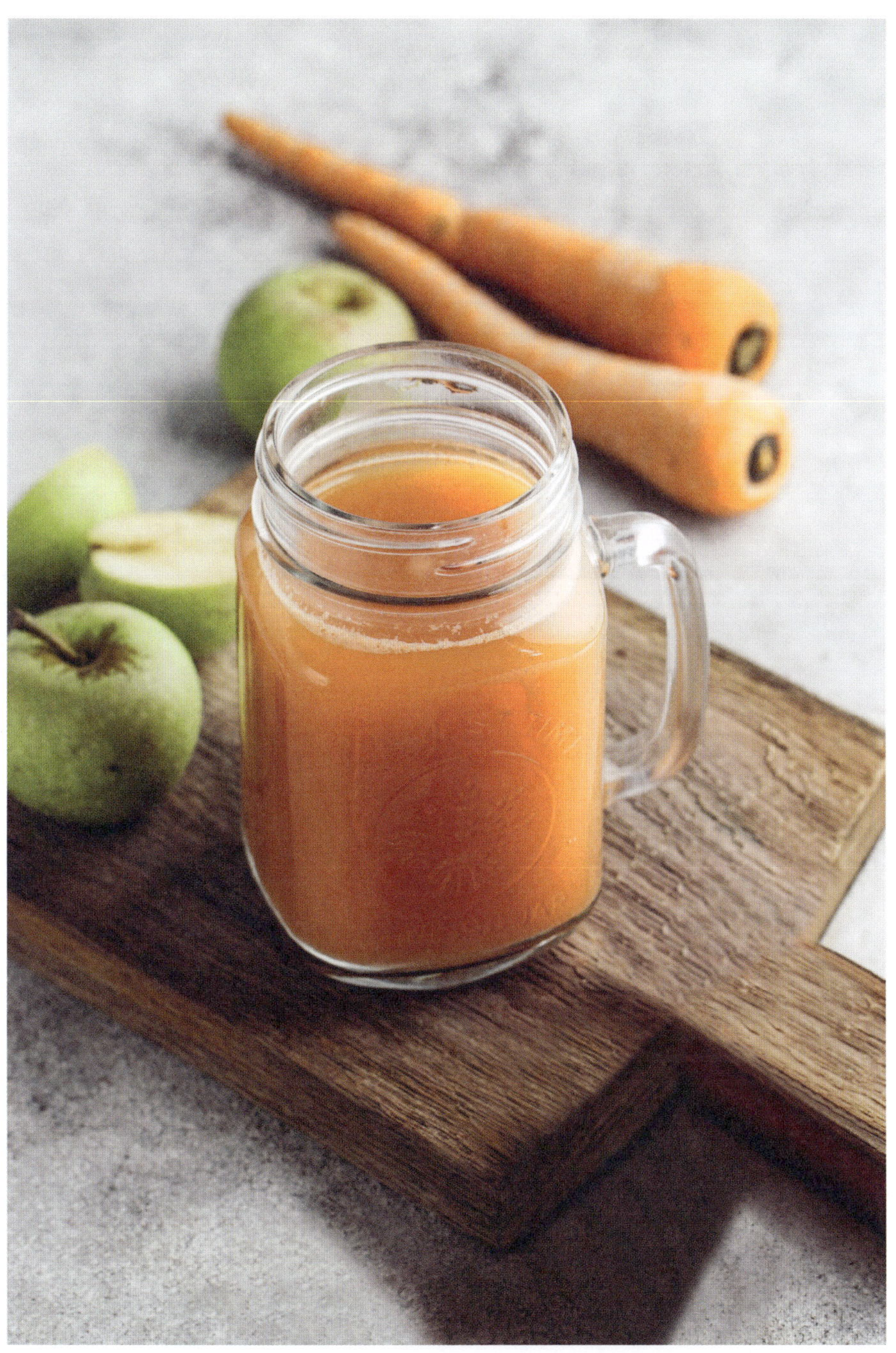

Pumpkin Spice Pancakes

Life can drag you in a million different directions each day, but you can stop the treadmill of insanity whenever you take a moment, connect to your breath, and choose to do what feels aligned with your soul and your highest good. Just like taking the time to make yourself pumpkin pancakes before a busy day can help you prioritize your joy, this meditation will help you choose to do the things you love.

YIELD: 2 servings

½ cup (120 ml) unsweetened almond milk
1 teaspoon cream of tartar
2 teaspoons flaxseed meal
2 tablespoons (30 ml) water (instead of flaxseed meal and water, you can use any vegan egg replacement for the equivalent of two eggs)
1 cup (148 g) gluten-free 1-to-1 flour
½ cup (123 g) pumpkin purée
2 tablespoons (30 ml) pumpkin pie spice (for homemade pumpkin pie spice, mix ½ teaspoon ground cinnamon, ⅛ teaspoon ground cloves, ¼ teaspoon ground ginger, and ⅛ teaspoon ground nutmeg)
2 tablespoons (30 ml) extra-virgin coconut oil
1 tablespoon (15 ml) vanilla extract
Coconut oil cooking spray, for greasing

FILLING (OPTIONAL)
8-ounce (237 g) container vegan cream cheese
2 tablespoons (30 ml) date (or maple) syrup
Sprinkle of ground nutmeg and cinnamon
Dash of vanilla extract

In a small cup, combine the almond milk and cream of tartar and set aside.

To make flax "egg," mix together the flaxseed and water in a small bowl and set aside for 5 minutes, until thickened.

In a medium mixing bowl, mix together the flour, pumpkin purée, pumpkin pie spice, coconut oil, vanilla extract, and the flax "egg."

Spray a medium frying pan or griddle pan with the cooking spray and heat over medium heat. Add the almond milk mixture to the mixing bowl and thoroughly mix. Pour 2 tablespoons of the batter into the pan and cook for 3 to 5 minutes, or until bubbles start to form and the edges begin to crisp. Flip and cook for another 30 seconds, and then transfer to a serving plate. Repeat with the remaining batter.

To make the filling, if using, combine all the filling ingredients in a stand mixer and beat until smooth and creamy. To serve, I love making silver dollar pancakes and stacking them with layers of the filling in between.

"

I choose to do things I love.

Meditation for the Positive Mind

Sit comfortably. Curl your ring finger and little finger into each palm with your thumbs holding them down, with your two standing fingers held together. Bring in your arms so that your elbows are by your sides and your hands are by your shoulders with the two standing fingers of each hand pointing straight up. Your forearms and hands should tilt forward slightly to an angle of 30 degrees from the vertical. Press your shoulders and elbows back and keep your palms facing forward. Close your eyes and focus them on your third-eye point (the space between your eyebrows). Take slow, deep breaths and mentally chant ***sa ta na ma*** from the third-eye point outward. This is a common Kundalini mantra that describes the cycle of life: ***sa*** means infinity, ***ta*** is life, ***na*** is death, and ***ma*** is rebirth. Start by practicing for 11 minutes, gradually building up to 31 minutes. Take a deep breath in to close, hold it, and then exhale and relax.

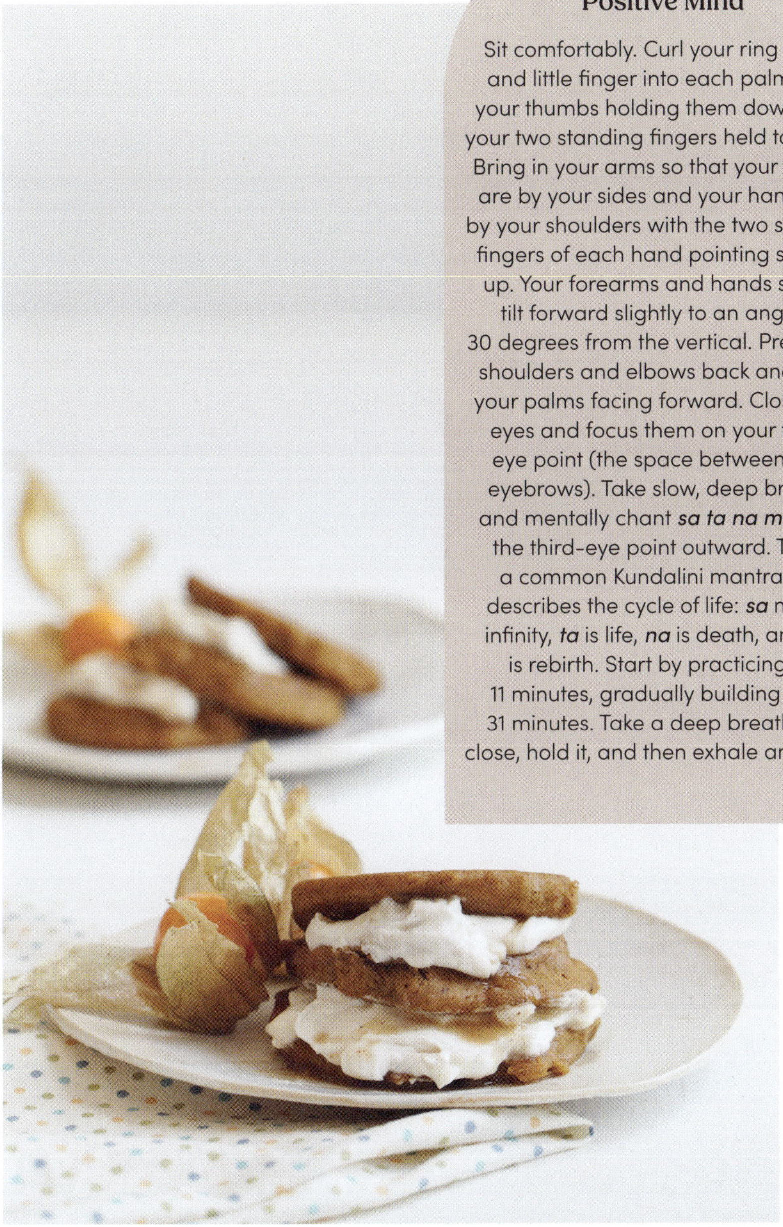

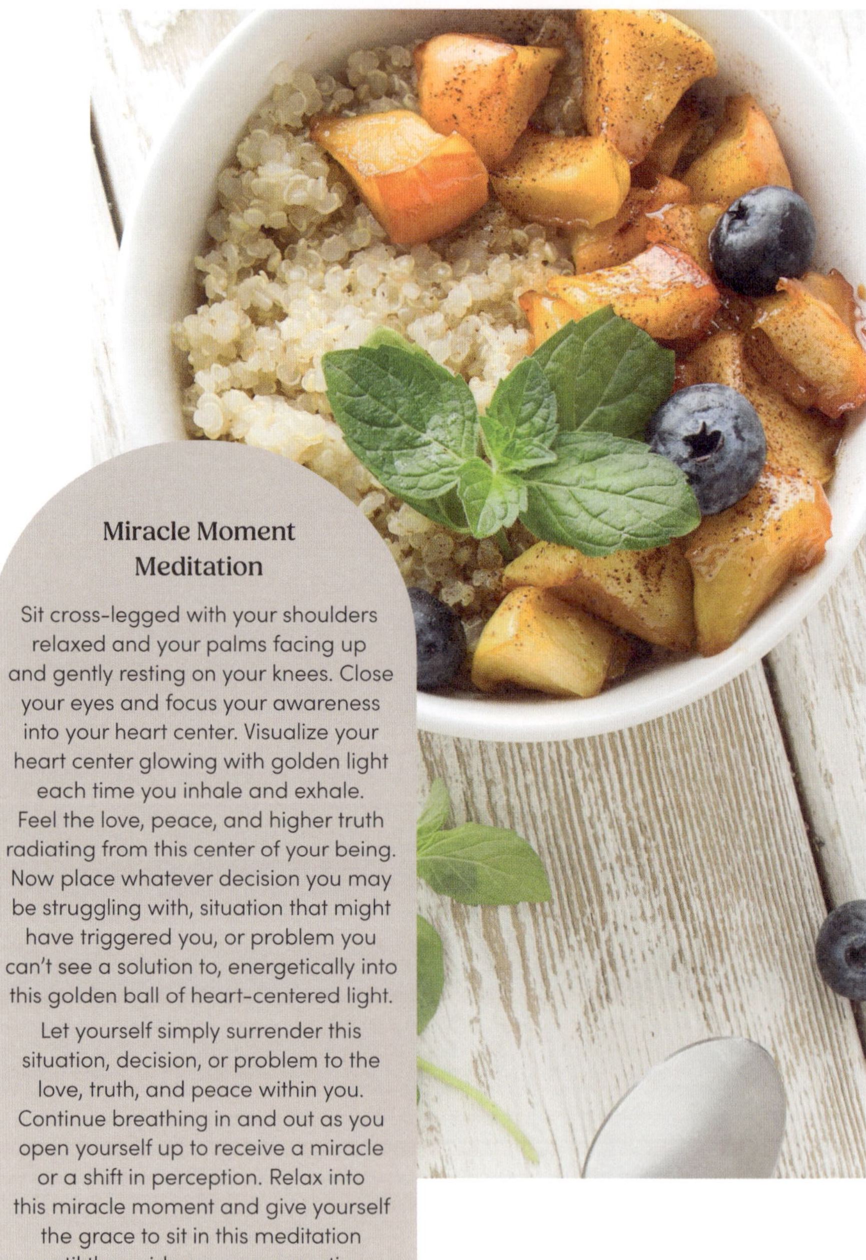

Miracle Moment Meditation

Sit cross-legged with your shoulders relaxed and your palms facing up and gently resting on your knees. Close your eyes and focus your awareness into your heart center. Visualize your heart center glowing with golden light each time you inhale and exhale. Feel the love, peace, and higher truth radiating from this center of your being. Now place whatever decision you may be struggling with, situation that might have triggered you, or problem you can't see a solution to, energetically into this golden ball of heart-centered light.

Let yourself simply surrender this situation, decision, or problem to the love, truth, and peace within you. Continue breathing in and out as you open yourself up to receive a miracle or a shift in perception. Relax into this miracle moment and give yourself the grace to sit in this meditation until the guidance or perspective you need emerges.

Quinoa Porridge

I like to refer to those few seconds when we have to decide how we want to react to something as the "miracle moment." When we anchor ourselves in a daily meditation practice, we give ourselves the space—that miracle moment—to see the options in front of us. Once we allow ourselves the space to think before we decide how to act, we step into our power around our responses. This warm, nourishing porridge feels like oatmeal but is loaded with a lot more protein thanks to our friend quinoa. It's the perfect way to ground yourself before a hectic day.

YIELD: 1 serving

- 1 cup (185 g) cooked quinoa
- 1 cup (237 ml) unsweetened vanilla coconut milk
- 1 peach (or any seasonal fruit), cut into small chunks
- ½ banana, sliced
- 3 tablespoons (27 g) chia seeds
- ¼ cup (18 g) sliced almonds (or nut/seed of your choice)
- ¼ cup (40 g) hemp hearts (optional topping)

In a small saucepan, combine the quinoa, coconut milk, and a little more than half of the peaches and banana and heat over medium-low heat. Add the chia seeds and stir continuously for 4 to 5 minutes, or until the mixture thickens and almost reaches a boil. Remove from the heat and set aside.

Transfer the quinoa porridge to a bowl, add the sliced almonds, hemp hearts, and remaining fruit, and then serve!

NOTE:
You can make this as a cold porridge by combining all the ingredients in a mason jar and leaving the jar in the fridge overnight for a cooling breakfast treat in the warmer months. You'll also have a filling breakfast ready for you on a busy morning!

PUMP UP THE PROTEIN:
Supplement the protein-packed quinoa by tossing more hemp hearts on top or mixing a scoop of your favorite vanilla plant-based protein powder into the porridge.

"

I allow myself the space to think before deciding.

Veggie Scramble with Turmeric Potatoes

When we take care of ourselves, we create a momentum that allows the universe to take care of us as well. This veggie scramble quickly became one of my go-to breakfasts once I started a plant-based diet and still wanted the "feel" and heartiness of my old scrambled eggs with potatoes.

YIELD: 2 servings

5 small fingerling (or new) potatoes, sliced into ¼-inch-thick (6 mm) rounds
2 tablespoons (30 ml) extra-virgin olive oil, divided
1 teaspoon ground turmeric
1 teaspoon garlic powder
1 teaspoon onion powder
1 teaspoon dried oregano
1 white onion, diced
1 clove to 1 bulb garlic, cloves separated, peeled, and chopped (amount depends on your taste)
½ zucchini, sliced
2 cups (220 g) leafy greens (I like a blend of baby kale, spinach, and bok choy)
½ cup (32 g) enoki mushrooms
½ avocado, halved, pitted, and sliced

Preheat the oven to 425°F (220°C, or gas mark 7).

In a small bowl, combine the potatoes, 1 tablespoon (15 ml) olive oil, turmeric, garlic powder, onion powder, and oregano and toss well. Pour the potatoes onto a baking sheet and roast for 10 minutes.

Meanwhile, heat the remaining 1 tablespoon (15 ml) olive oil in a medium frying pan over medium heat. Add the onion and garlic, stir for 1 to 2 minutes, and then add the zucchini. Cook for another 5 minutes, until golden and tender. Add the leafy greens and continue to stir until the greens are bright green and wilted. Transfer the mixture to a serving plate.

Check on the potatoes and if they have started to brown, remove them from the oven and let them cool on the stovetop. If they still have a few minutes to go, leave them in while you finish up the last few steps.

In the same frying pan (no need to clean), heat the mushrooms over medium heat and fry until browned. Place the mushrooms on top of the vegetable mixture. Serve the roasted potatoes on the side and top it all off with sliced avocado!

PUMP UP THE PROTEIN:
Simply add the tofu scramble from the Brunch Tacos recipe (page 39) to get some additional protein into this meal.

"
I honor my basic needs.

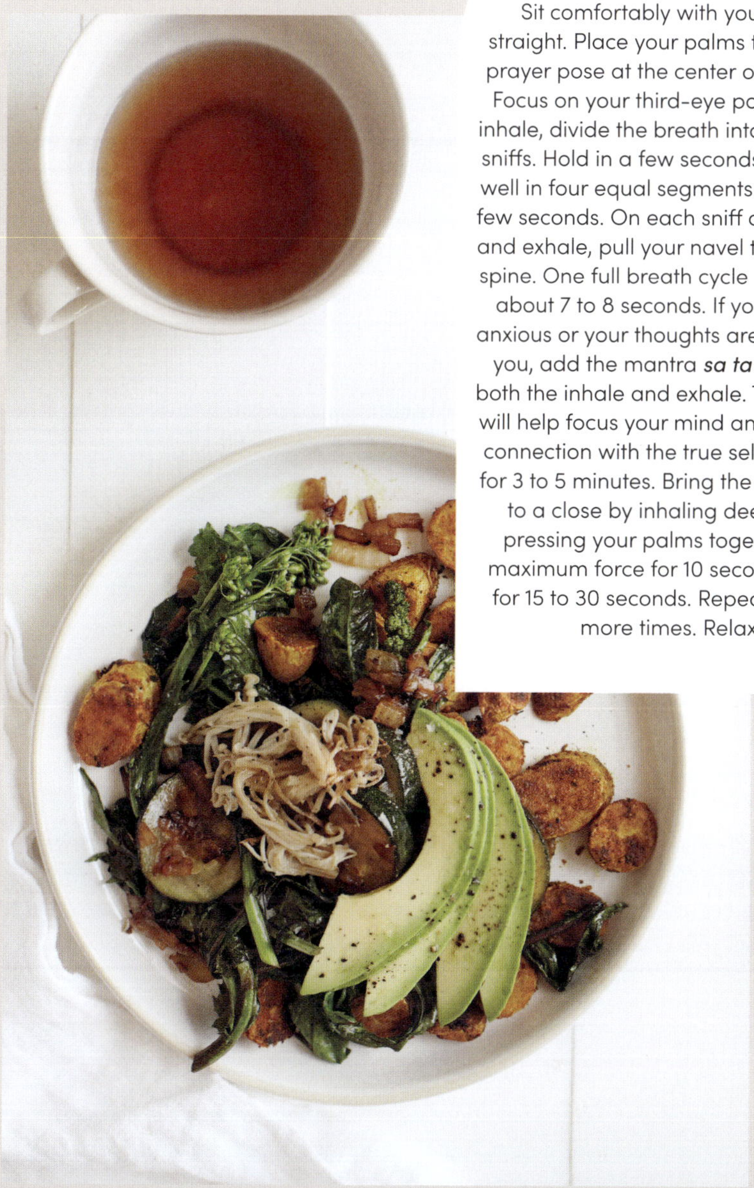

Meditation for Increased Energy

Sit comfortably with your spine straight. Place your palms together in prayer pose at the center of the chest. Focus on your third-eye point. As you inhale, divide the breath into four equal sniffs. Hold in a few seconds. Exhale as well in four equal segments. Hold out a few seconds. On each sniff of the inhale and exhale, pull your navel toward your spine. One full breath cycle should take about 7 to 8 seconds. If your mind is anxious or your thoughts are distracting you, add the mantra ***sa ta na ma*** on both the inhale and exhale. This mantra will help focus your mind and stimulate connection with the true self. Continue for 3 to 5 minutes. Bring the meditation to a close by inhaling deeply and pressing your palms together with maximum force for 10 seconds. Relax for 15 to 30 seconds. Repeat this two more times. Relax.

Cauliflower Apple Rosemary Soup

Whenever I feel my patience running low, I think about the acorn growing into an oak tree and remind myself that my patience allows the magic to happen—I can trust that if I've planted the seed, nature will make the flower blossom. As you follow the different steps of making this soup, you can slow down and enjoy the prepping, roasting, and blending, trusting that it will come together in it's time for this delicious dish.

And when you need extra assistance, the meditation will help you release any negative thoughts getting in the way of enjoying the present moment.

YIELD: 4 servings

Olive oil cooking spray, for greasing
1 head cauliflower, chopped
2 teaspoons garlic powder
2 teaspoons onion powder
Salt and freshly ground black pepper, to taste
2 apples, thinly sliced (I prefer Pink Lady apples)
2 tablespoons (30 ml) extra-virgin olive oil
1 white onion, diced
1 clove garlic, chopped
3 cups (720 g) unsweetened almond milk, divided (substitute mushroom or veggie broth if you want a lighter or nut-free version)
3 tablespoons (45 g) Dijon mustard
4 rosemary sprigs, divided

"

My patience is precious.

Preheat the oven to 425°F (220°C, or gas mark 7). Grease a baking sheet with cooking spray. Add the cauliflower, sprinkle over the garlic and onion powders, and generously season with salt and pepper. Roast in the oven for 10 to 15 minutes, or until the cauliflower starts to brown.

In the meantime, grease another baking sheet with cooking spray and scatter the apples across it. Bake for 5 minutes, or until the apples begin to brown.

Heat the olive oil in a frying pan over medium heat. Add the onion and sauté for 5 minutes until softened, then add the garlic and sauté for another minute.

Transfer the roasted cauliflower and apples (setting aside a few apple slices to garnish) to a food processor or high-speed blender, and then add the onions and garlic, 1 cup (240 ml) almond milk, and Dijon mustard. Pulse until puréed, gradually adding more almond milk to achieve your desired consistency.

Transfer the mixture into a large saucepan over medium heat, add 2 rosemary sprigs, and simmer for 10 minutes until warm and infused with rosemary. Remove the rosemary.

To serve, finely chop the remaining rosemary leaves. Ladle the soup into individual bowls, and then garnish with sliced apples and chopped rosemary.

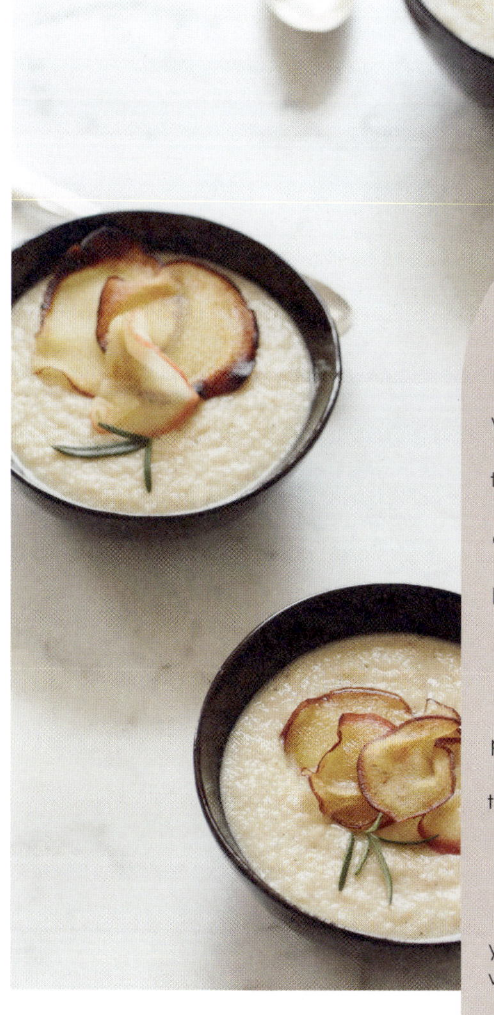

Kundalini Meditation for the Negative Mind

Sit comfortably. Make a cup with your hands, right inside of left, with both palms facing up. Close your eyes most of the way, and look down toward your cupped hands. Place this open cup at the level of your heart center and allow your elbows to relax at your sides. Inhale deeply, taking a long, steady breath through the nose. Exhale in a focused stream through rounded lips, as if you were blowing a feather out of your hands. Let any thought or desire that is negative or persistently distracting come into your mind as you breathe. Breathe the thought in, then exhale it out. Continue for 11 minutes, gradually building to 31 minutes. Close by inhaling completely and then exhaling and holding the breath out as you lock in your navel point. Concentrate on each vertebra of the spine until you can feel it all the way to the base, as if it is as stiff as a rod. Inhale powerfully, exhale completely. Repeat this final action 3 to 5 times, then relax completely.

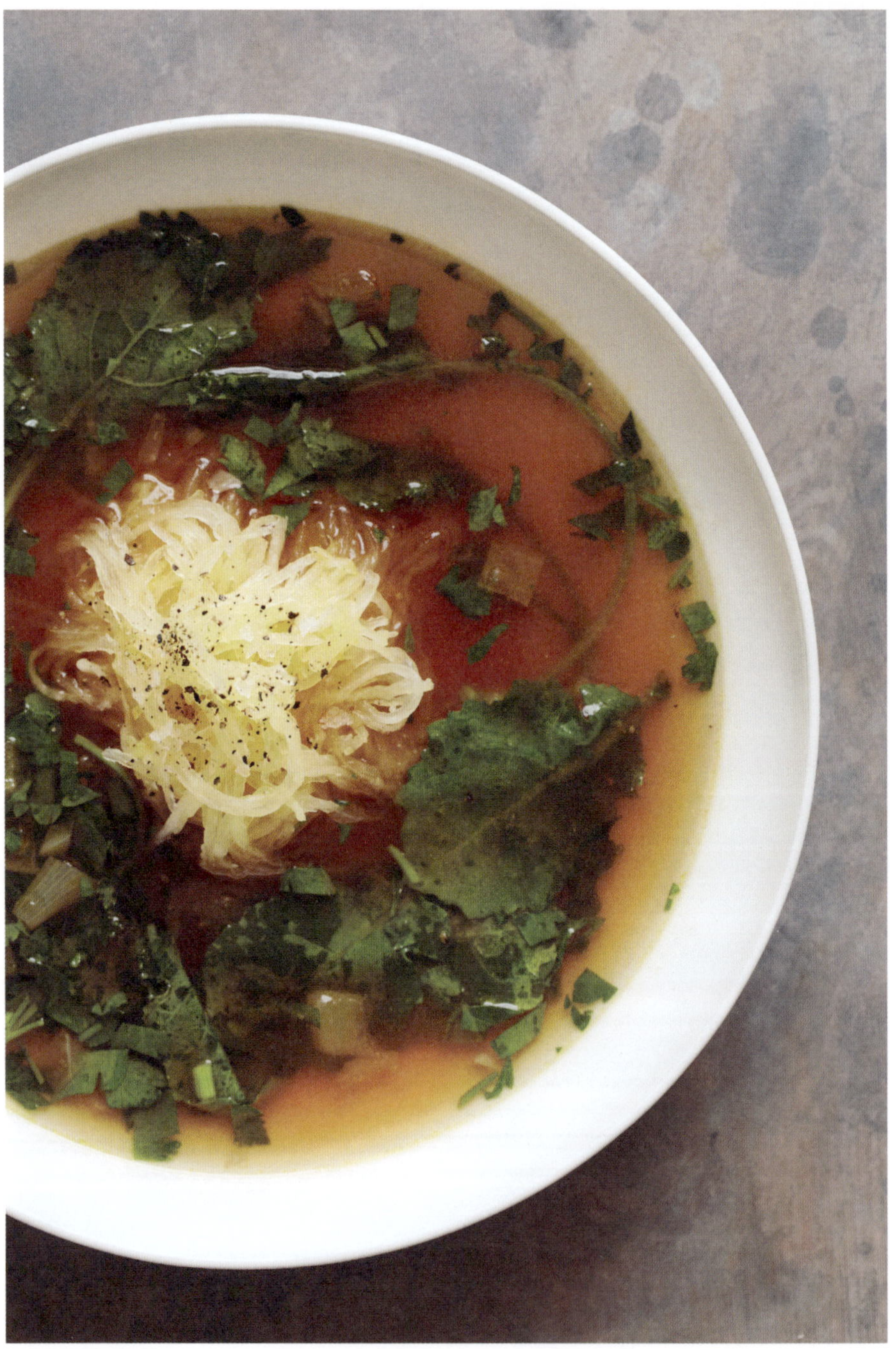

Spaghetti Squash Noodle Soup

When we spend our time worrying about the future or ruminating on the past, we are not only unhappy, we are also not really living! Getting present is the most basic, life-changing adjustment you can commit to. The thing I love about making this soup is that it commands you to settle into the moment, stirring, smelling its sweet aroma.

YIELD: 4 servings

1 spaghetti squash, halved lengthwise
2 tablespoons (30 ml) extra-virgin olive oil, divided
1 onion, diced
1 clove garlic, chopped
4 cups (960 ml) vegetable or mushroom broth
2 cups (136 g) baby spinach
2 tablespoons (8 g) chopped fresh parsley
2 tablespoons (4 g) chopped fresh oregano
Salt and freshly ground black pepper, to taste

Preheat the oven to 425°F (220°C, or gas mark 7).

Brush the inside of the spaghetti squash with 1 tablespoon (15 ml) olive oil and lay them, facing down, on a medium baking sheet. Roast for 40 minutes, or until softened.

Scoop out the seeds and discard. Use a fork to scrape out the "spaghetti" strings and transfer to a bowl.

Heat the remaining 1 tablespoon (15 ml) olive oil in a large frying pan over medium heat. Add the onions and sauté for 5 minutes until softened, then add the garlic and sauté for another minute. Put in the spaghetti squash and cook for another 5 minutes. Pour in the vegetable broth, add the baby spinach, parsley, and oregano, and stir until well mixed.

Bring to a boil, reduce the heat, and simmer for 10 minutes, until thoroughly warmed. Season with salt and pepper to taste.

A Living Meditation

A living meditation is a practice to employ all the time to make your daily experience as blissful as possible, but a lot of us are so out of touch with being present these days that it helps to begin in small doses. I encourage you to try this practice daily and transition it into a way of life. Begin by setting a timer for 30 minutes. Take a deep breath in and get really present with what is right in front of you. Maybe you are making this soup, maybe you are drinking tea and sitting on your couch; whatever it is, take it in with all five senses. Pay attention to the sound of the birds outside your window, smell the squash as it comes out of the oven, enjoy the taste of each sip of tea. Be here now. And when a thought comes up that wants to distract you with what's going on later today or tomorrow, take a deep breath and bring yourself right back here, to the now.

"

I find the presents in the present.

Spicy Squash Soup

How often do we let one little mistake send us off the deep end? When we are having trouble processing our feelings, we may also have trouble with our digestion. This soothing soup's little kick of spice will help you keep moving forward!

YIELD: 4 servings

2 tablespoons (24 g) raw extra-virgin coconut oil
1 acorn squash, halved lengthwise and seeded (a smaller butternut squash works as well)
2 red peppers, seeded and coarsely chopped
2 tablespoons (30 ml) extra-virgin olive oil
1 onion, diced
1 clove garlic, chopped
2 cups (480 ml) vegetable broth
½ teaspoon chili powder
½ teaspoon ground cumin
½ teaspoon ground coriander
½ teaspoon curry powder
½ teaspoon paprika
½ teaspoon ground turmeric
Salt and freshly ground black pepper, to taste

Preheat the oven to 425°F (220°C, or gas mark 7). Grease 2 medium baking sheets with coconut oil.

Slice 1 inch (2.5 cm) from the bottom of each acorn squash so that they sit flat on a prepared baking sheet. Scatter the peppers on the other baking sheet. Roast both for 20 minutes, until the squash has softened and the peppers get color. Set aside.

Meanwhile, heat the olive oil in a large frying pan over medium heat. Add the onions and sauté for 5 minutes until softened, then add the garlic and sauté for another minute. Transfer the mixture to a high-speed blender or food processor, and then add the vegetable broth and spices.

Once the squashes are cool enough to handle, trim off the skin from each and cut both into chunks. Add the squash and peppers to the blender or food processor and purée until smooth and creamy.

Season with salt and pepper, transfer the soup to a saucepan, and heat over medium heat until warmed through. Serve.

"

I give myself a clean slate through forgiveness.

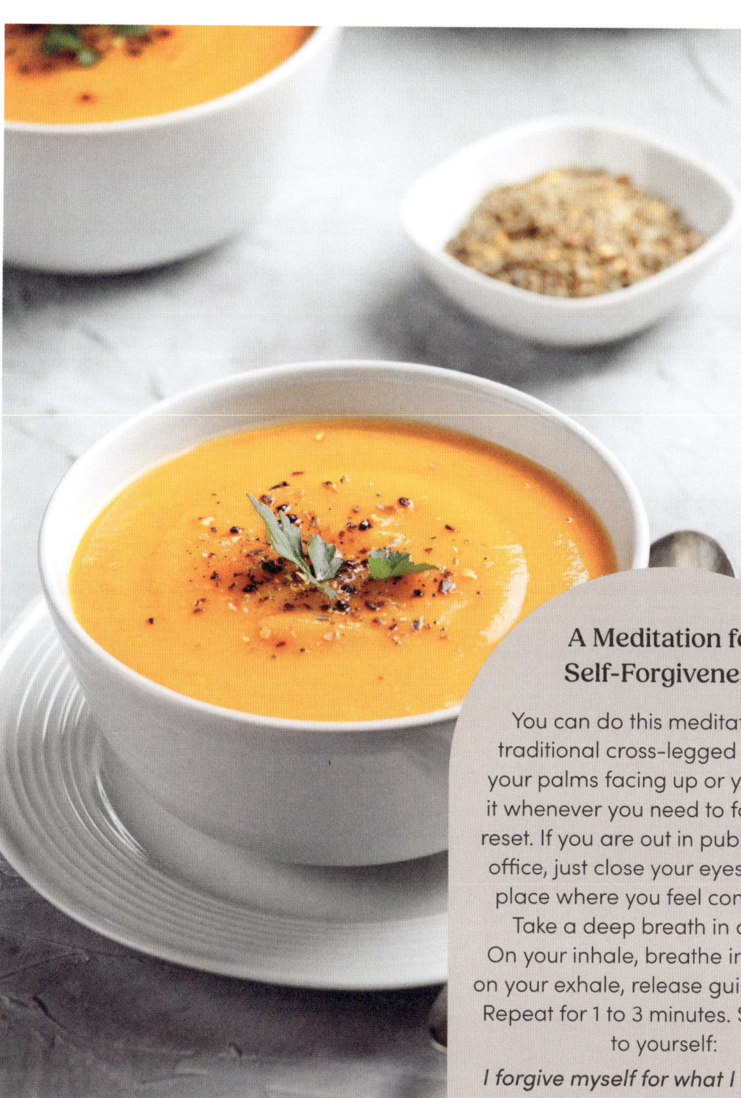

A Meditation for Self-Forgiveness

You can do this meditation in a traditional cross-legged seat with your palms facing up or you can do it whenever you need to forgive and reset. If you are out in public or at the office, just close your eyes in a quiet place where you feel comfortable. Take a deep breath in and out. On your inhale, breathe in love, and on your exhale, release guilt or shame. Repeat for 1 to 3 minutes. Silently say to yourself:

I forgive myself for what I have done and choose to do better. I choose to begin again with a clean slate.

Take a deep breath in and hold it, filling yourself up with love and forgiveness, exhale, and relax. Repeat as often as necessary if feelings of guilt, shame, or "ruining it" come up.

Grounding Salad

By connecting back to nature and eating more root vegetables and warm foods, we bring ourselves back to a steady, more-powerful place. This salad not only quenches the desire for fresh greens, but it also includes hearty roasted veggies, such as brussels sprouts, carrots, and potatoes, along with lots of great spices, to bring you back down into your root chakra.

YIELD: 2 servings

5 tablespoons (75 ml) extra-virgin olive oil, divided
4 baby potatoes, sliced (I prefer the colored ones but any kind will do!)
1 teaspoon dried oregano
2 teaspoons fine sea salt, divided
2 teaspoons garlic powder, divided
2 teaspoons onion powder, divided
½ cup (44 g) quartered brussels sprouts
1 clove garlic, thinly sliced
1 shallot, thinly sliced
¼ cup (31 g) sliced carrot
2 teaspoons slivered almonds
1 teaspoon ground turmeric
1 teaspoon curry powder
1 teaspoon ground coriander
1 cup (68 g) chopped kale, spinach, or arugula
1 cup (29 g) spring mix salad

GET CREATIVE:
The beauty of this salad is really in the combination of the warm roasted vegetables and the fresh bed of greens. Feel free to experiment with whatever veggies you have available or try new things you find at the farmers market! Beets, sweet potatoes, sunchokes, and artichoke hearts are also fabulous in this recipe.

Preheat the oven to 425°F (220°C, or gas mark 7). Lightly grease 2 baking sheets with 2 tablespoons (30 ml) olive oil and set aside.

In a small bowl, combine the potatoes, oregano, 1 tablespoon (15 ml) olive oil, and 1 teaspoon each of the salt, garlic, and onion powder and mix until thoroughly coated. Transfer the potatoes to one of the prepared baking sheets and roast for 10 minutes, or until the edges turn crisp and golden brown.

Meanwhile, combine the brussels sprouts and 1 tablespoon (15 ml) olive oil in a small bowl and toss with the remaining 1 teaspoon salt, garlic powder, and onion powder. Arrange them on the other prepared baking sheet and roast in the oven for 5 to 7 minutes, or until the edges turn crisp and golden brown.

Heat the remaining 1 tablespoon (15 ml) olive oil in a frying pan over medium heat. Add the garlic and shallot and sauté for 1 minute until fragrant. Add the sliced carrots, almonds, turmeric, curry powder, and ground coriander, reduce the heat, and lightly sauté for several minutes, until the shallots and garlic are browned.

Divide the kale and spring mix between 2 individual serving bowls. Add the roasted potatoes and brussels sprouts, and then finish with the carrot mixture.

“

I am grounded and steady.

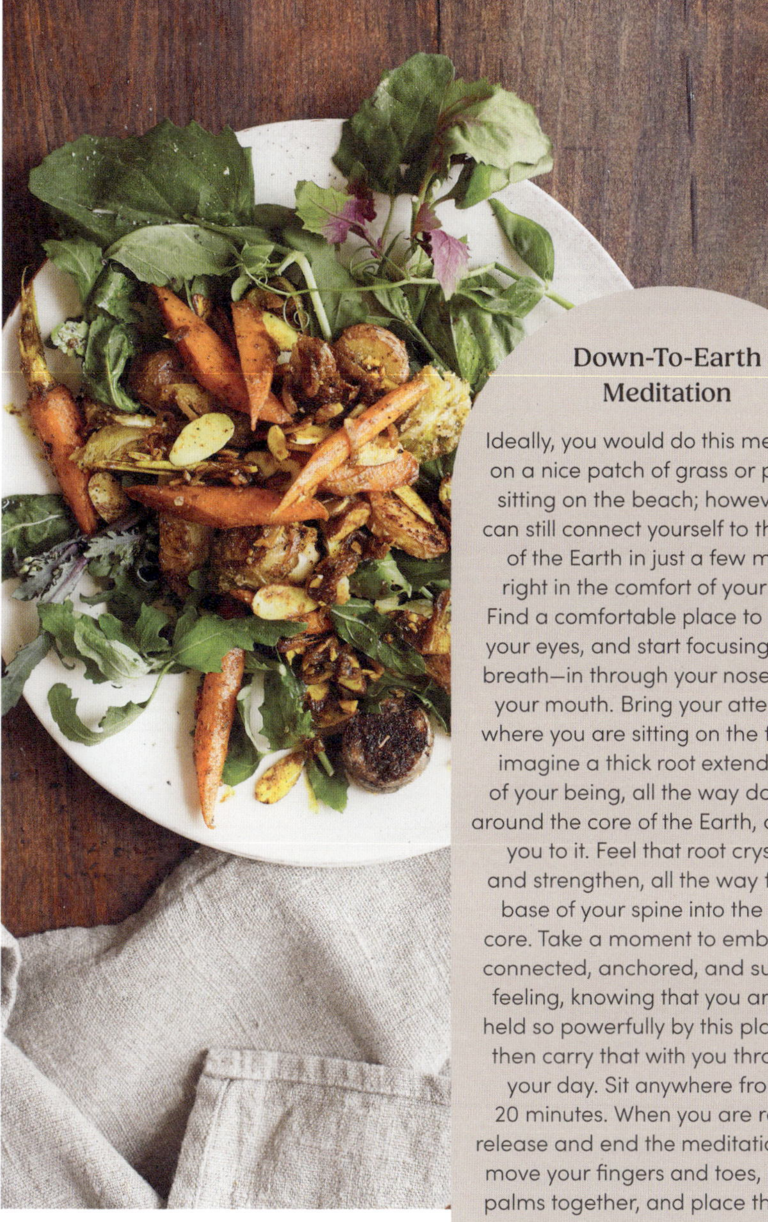

Down-To-Earth Meditation

Ideally, you would do this meditation on a nice patch of grass or perhaps sitting on the beach; however, you can still connect yourself to the center of the Earth in just a few minutes right in the comfort of your home. Find a comfortable place to sit, close your eyes, and start focusing on your breath—in through your nose and out your mouth. Bring your attention to where you are sitting on the floor and imagine a thick root extending out of your being, all the way down and around the core of the Earth, anchoring you to it. Feel that root crystallize and strengthen, all the way from the base of your spine into the Earth's core. Take a moment to embrace this connected, anchored, and supported feeling, knowing that you are being held so powerfully by this planet, and then carry that with you throughout your day. Sit anywhere from 3 to 20 minutes. When you are ready to release and end the meditation, gently move your fingers and toes, rub your palms together, and place them over your eye sockets as you slowly open your eyes and expose them to the light.

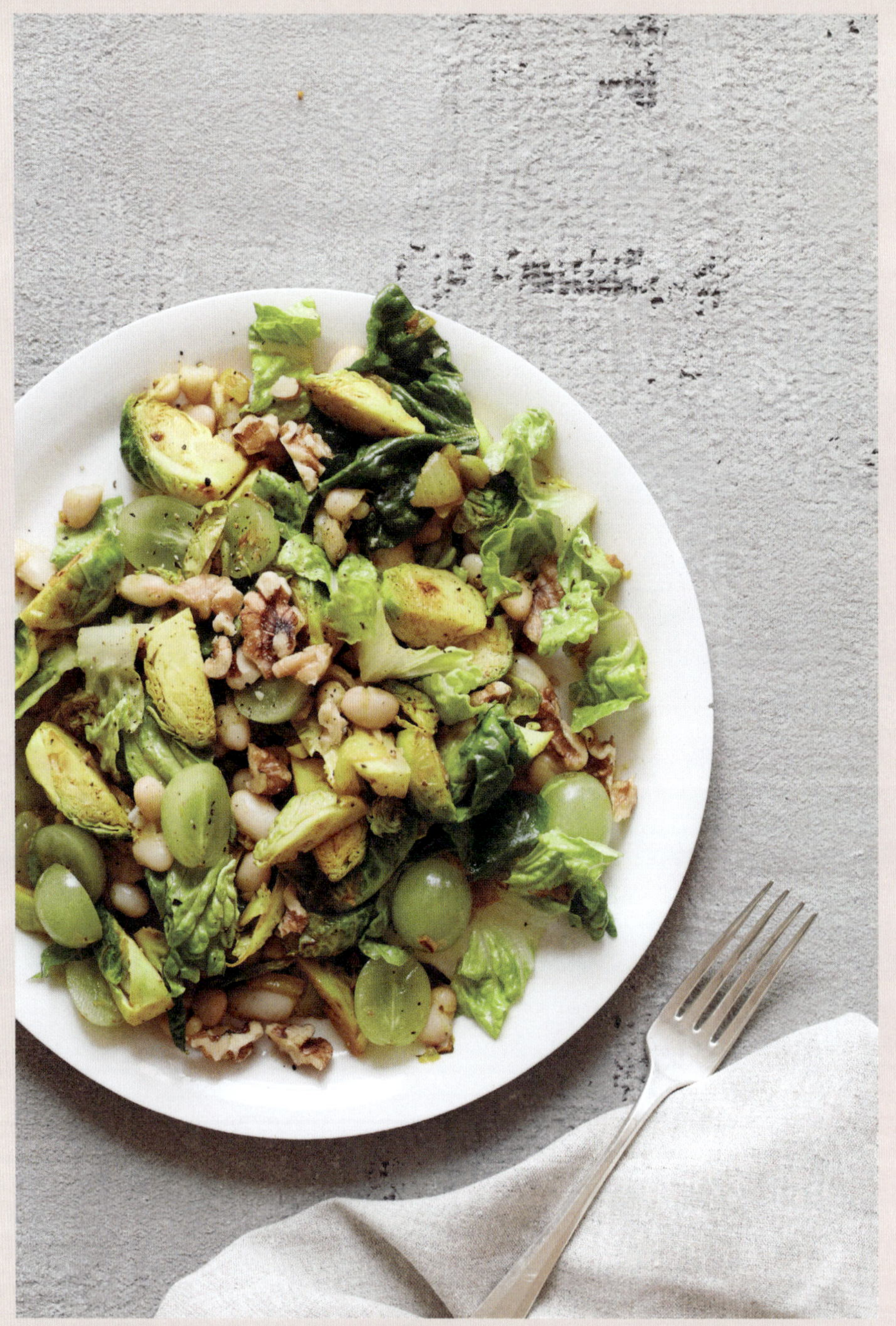

Shaved Brussels Sprout Salad

Your excuses are weighing you down, but, at any moment, you can decide to step into your power. Growing up, I had a strong resistance to brussels sprouts. My mom used to boil them and call them "Martian heads", which made me detest them even more. As an adult, I made a decision to make these Martian heads delicious, and now I'm a full-blown addict.

YIELD: 2 servings

2 tablespoons (30 ml) extra-virgin olive oil
½ onion, diced
1 clove garlic, finely chopped
2 cups (176 g) quartered brussels sprouts
1 teaspoon ground turmeric
1 teaspoon garlic powder
1 teaspoon onion powder
Salt and freshly ground black pepper, to taste
½ head romaine lettuce, chopped
1 cup (260 g) cannellini beans, rinsed and drained
1 cup (151 g) sliced grapes
2 tablespoons (13 g) chopped walnuts, to garnish

Heat the oil in a large saucepan over medium heat. Add the onions and sauté for 5 minutes until softened, then add the garlic and sauté for another minute. Add the brussels sprouts, turmeric, garlic powder, and onion powder, and mix well. Season with salt and pepper to taste, then reduce the heat to low and set aside to continue cooking.

Combine the lettuce, cannellini beans, and grapes in a large bowl. Add the brussels sprout mixture and toss well. Place in individual serving bowls and garnish with the walnuts.

Meditation for Releasing Excuses

Find a comfortable place to sit with your palms facing up and your eyes closed. Take a deep breath in through your nose and exhale out your mouth. Feel the breath moving through your body. Notice where in your body you are tight or knotted up and breathe into that spot; allow the tightness to release with each exhale. Now bring to mind a situation in which you have been making a lot of excuses and ask to see it clearly. Honor anything that might come up around this situation. Allow any and all excuses you have been making to come to the forefront of your mind, inhaling the excuse, exhaling and tossing it out of your mind and into the air. Repeat until you find yourself running out of excuses. Return to the original situation and ask to see it clearly. Sit and take a few long, deep breaths. Honor what you see or hear in this moment. When you are ready, take a deep breath in and hold it, then exhale and relax.

"

I release my excuses and step into my power.

Tomato Arugula Salad

I love this salad because of its simplicity. When you are eating fresh, nutrient-dense food, you don't have to do much to it. You can just let it shine.

YIELD: 4 servings

3 cups (525 g) couscous
3 cups (711 ml) water
4 cups (80 g) arugula
1 cup (149 g) grape tomatoes, halved
1 cucumber, peeled and diced
½ red onion, diced
½ cup black olives, halved
2 tablespoons (4 g) chopped fresh oregano
2 tablespoons (6 g) chopped fresh basil
Juice of 1 lemon
3 tablespoons (45 ml) balsamic vinegar
5 tablespoons (75 ml) extra-virgin olive oil, divided
Salt and freshly ground black pepper, to taste
½ cup vegan feta cheese crumbles (optional)

Put the couscous and water in a medium saucepan and bring to a boil. Reduce the heat and simmer, covered, for 10 minutes or until cooked through.

Fluff the couscous with a fork. In a large bowl, combine the arugula, couscous, tomatoes, cucumber, red onion, olives, oregano, and basil. Mix well.

Combine the lemon juice, balsamic vinegar, and olive oil, and drizzle it over the couscous and veggies. Season with salt and pepper to taste, transfer to a platter, sprinkle with feta if desired, and serve.

Basic Breath

The basics start with your breath. Use this whenever or wherever you are as a simple tool to bring you back home, especially in moments of overwhelm.

Close your eyes and relax your face and your shoulders. Take a deep breath in through your nose and out your mouth and just focus your attention on the breath. Allow any thoughts that come up to pass by, returning your attention to your breath. Feel the breath circulate throughout your entire being as it goes in your nose and out your mouth. Continue for 3 minutes or as long as you want.

"

When I get overwhelmed, I go back to basics.

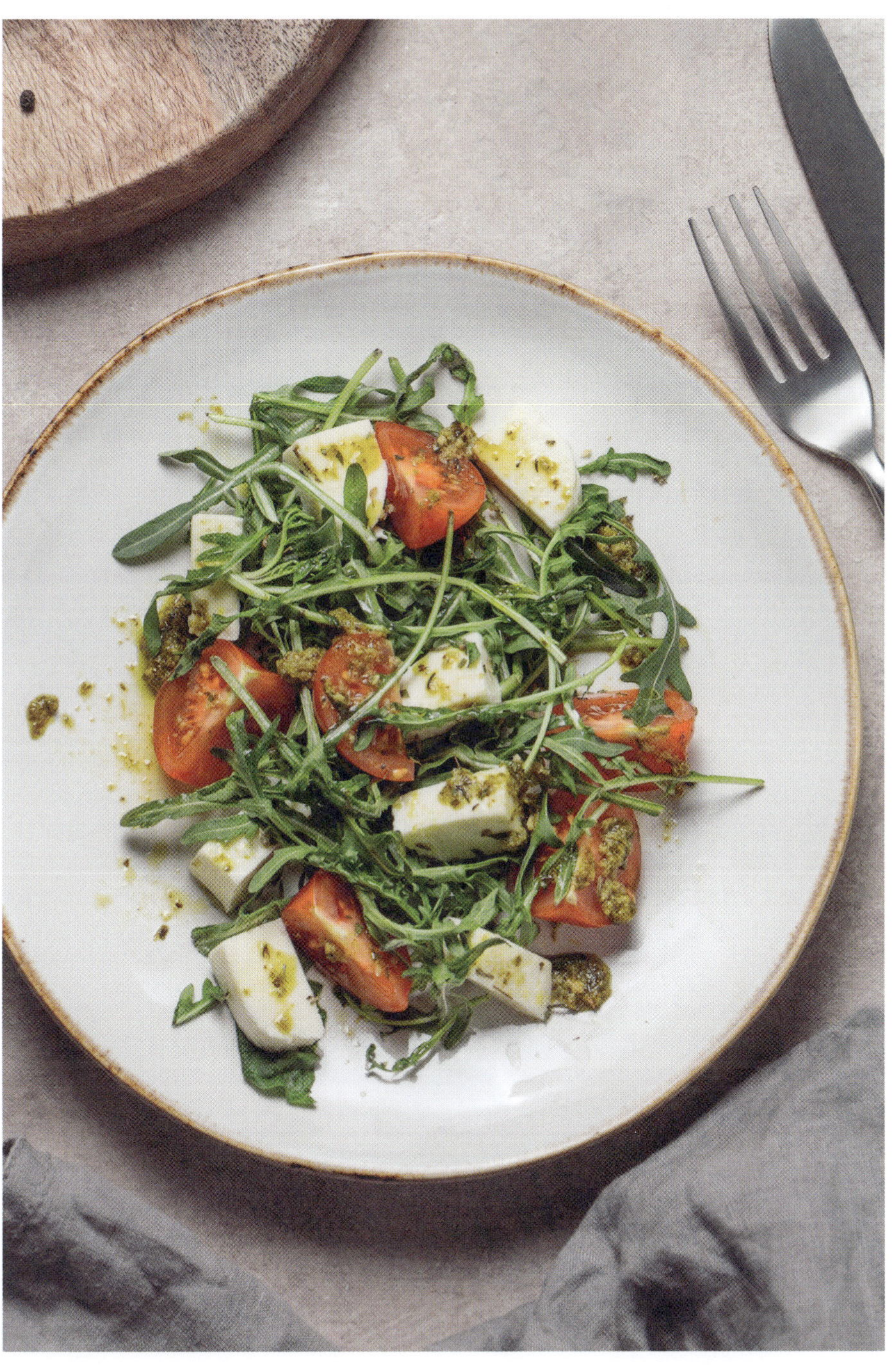

Cauliflower Fried Rice

A miracle can be as simple as a shift in perspective. This dish is a great example of seeing things differently: It turns out, fried rice doesn't have to be made with rice at all. Here, I turned cauliflower into "rice" in my food processor. Also, it's absolutely delicious.

YIELD: 2 servings

1 head cauliflower, florets separated and coarsely chopped
1 tablespoon (15 ml) sesame oil
1 yellow onion, diced
1 clove garlic, chopped
2 cups (170 g) broccoli slaw (with cabbage and carrots)
2 tablespoons (18 g) sesame seeds
½ cup (50 g) chopped scallions

SAUCE
¼ cup (80 ml) tamari (gluten-free soy sauce)
2-inch (5 cm) piece ginger root, finely chopped (use less if you are not a huge fan of ginger)
1 tablespoon (15 ml) onion powder

Place the cauliflower in a food processor and pulse until rice-like in appearance. Set aside.

Heat the sesame oil in a large frying pan over medium heat, add the onion, garlic, and broccoli slaw, and sauté for 2 minutes.

To make the sauce, combine the ingredients in a small bowl and mix well.

Stir the cauliflower rice into the broccoli-slaw mixture, and then add the sesame seeds and sauce. Cook for another 5 minutes, and then transfer into individual serving bowls and top with the chopped scallions.

PUMP UP THE PROTEIN:
If you want to make an even heartier version of this recipe, add the tofu scramble from the brunch taco recipe on page 39.

Asking for a Miracle

Close your eyes, if possible. Put your hands on your heart, and bring to the top of your mind the situation for which you are asking for a miracle. Once you have it, simply say,

I surrender this situation. I am willing to see things differently. I am ready for a miracle. Thank you.

Take a deep breath in and feel that miracle on its way and then exhale. Relax and go about your day. If the situation pops up again throughout the day, simply repeat,

I surrender this situation. I am willing to see things differently.

Expect miracles!

"

I am willing to see things differently.

Mushroom Tacos

I love this dish because it offers a whole new experience of a taco. It reminds me that when I'm facing a new beginning, I have to let go of what I thought I knew and focus on what I can create moving forward.

YIELD: 4 tacos

Olive oil cooking spray, for greasing
6 new potatoes, diced
Sea salt, to taste
2 tablespoons (30 ml) extra-virgin olive oil
½ white onion, quartered
1 clove garlic, chopped
¾ cup (53 g) chopped cremini mushrooms
¾ cup (65 g) chopped oyster mushrooms
¾ cup (48 g) enoki mushrooms
4 corn tortillas (or gluten-free taco shells)
4 romaine lettuce leaves, roughly chopped

SAUCE
1 avocado, halved and pitted
2 or 3 sprigs cilantro
2 tablespoons (30 g) grated horseradish
2 tablespoons (28 g) vegan sour cream

Preheat the oven to 425°F (220°C, or gas mark 7).

Grease a medium baking sheet with cooking spray. Sprinkle the potatoes with salt and roast in the oven for 10 to 15 minutes, until they begin to brown.

Heat the oil in a large frying pan over medium heat. Add the onions and sauté for 3 minutes, or until softened, then add the garlic and sauté for another minute. Add the mushrooms and cook for 5 minutes.

To make the sauce, pulse the avocado, cilantro, horseradish, and sour cream in a food processor until thick and creamy.

Place a tortilla in a dry frying pan over medium heat and cook for about 45 seconds on each side, until warm and lightly brown. Repeat with the remaining tortillas.

To plate, lay out the warm tortillas. Place the chopped lettuce in the center, top with the mushroom mixture and roasted potatoes, and drizzle with the tangy avocado cream sauce. Enjoy!

Setting Intentions Visualization

Sit in a comfortable seated position with your palms facing up on your knees and your eyes closed. Take a few deep breaths and see yourself sitting on a blanket in front of a fertile garden plot with fresh soil. The sun warms your skin and you notice a small pile of seeds to your right. Pick up a seed and hold it in your hand. Set an intention for a new beginning, to create something in your life; see and feel what it looks like. When you are ready, dig a small hole in front of you and plant the seed. Repeat this as many times as you like. When you have planted your seeds, place both of your hands over the dirt and infuse it with love. Allow yourself to feel supported, knowing that your seeds are on their way to sprouting. Take a deep breath in and hold it, filling yourself up with gratitude and excitement for all these new beginnings, and then exhale.

"

I welcome a new beginning.

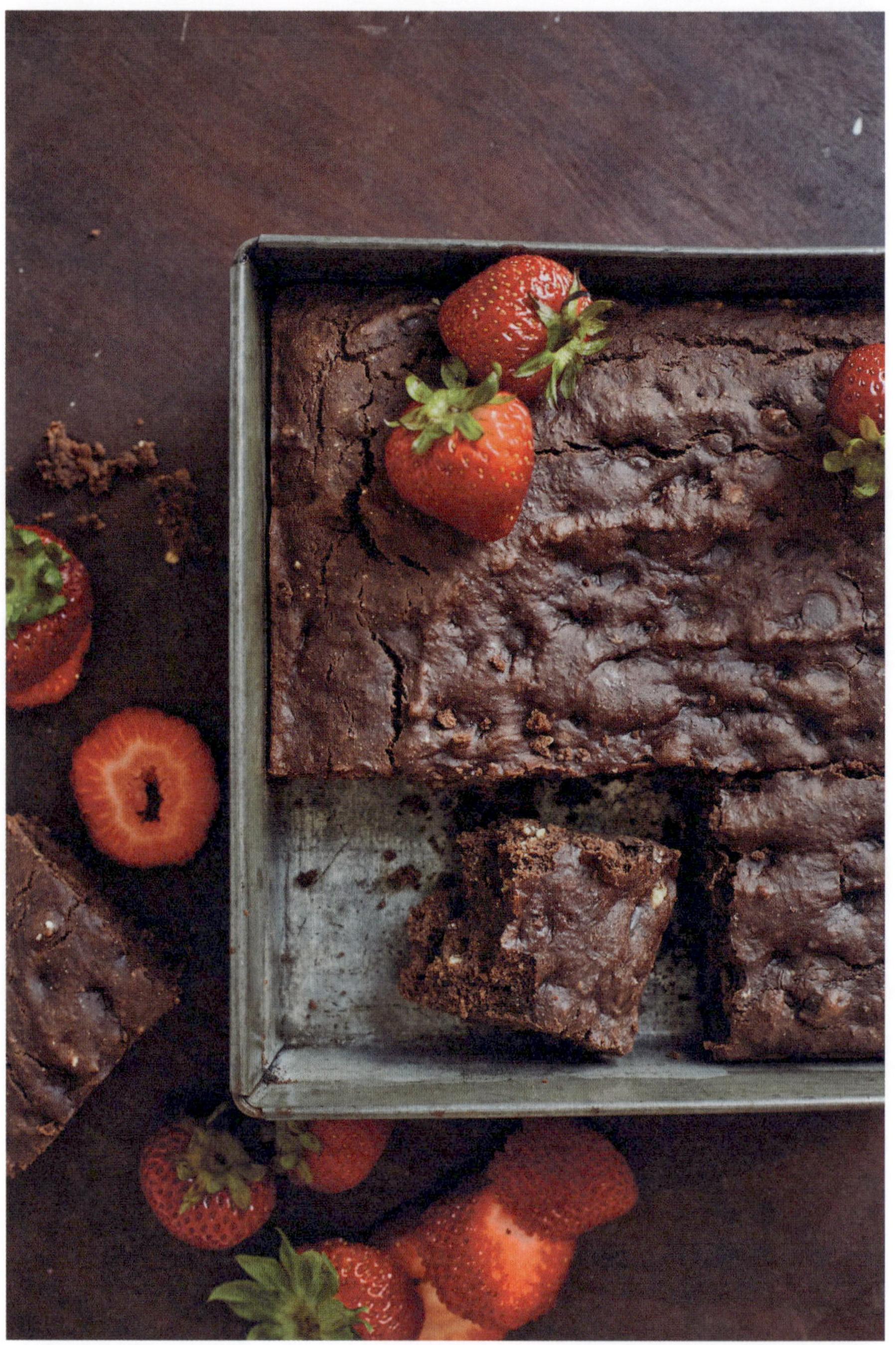

Barely Baked Brownies

Nothing reminds me more of the emotional disasters that have resulted from being too attached to something than indulging in a tray of brownies! Well, now you can eat these healthier brownies from a place of joy.

YIELD: 8 servings

2 teaspoons flaxseed meal
2 tablespoons (30 ml) water
1 tablespoon (12 g) raw extra-virgin coconut oil, for greasing
1 ⅓ cups (197 g) gluten-free 1-to-1 flour
1 cup (244 g) unsweetened applesauce
1 cup (224 g) vegan sugar-free chocolate chips
¾ cup (65 g) unsweetened cocoa powder
½ cup (120 ml) brown-rice syrup (or maple syrup)
1 teaspoon vanilla extract
½ teaspoon baking soda
Chopped walnuts, to garnish
Berries, to garnish

To make the flax "egg," mix together the flaxseed and water in a small bowl and set aside for 5 minutes, until thickened.

Preheat the oven to 375°F (190°C, or gas mark 5) and grease an 8-inch (20 cm) baking dish with coconut oil.

In a medium mixing bowl, combine all of the remaining ingredients (except the walnuts and berries) and flax "egg" until thoroughly mixed and pour the batter into the prepared baking dish.

Bake for 15 to 20 minutes and then remove to cool. (Cook for less time if you really want them "barely baked.")

Garnish with chopped walnuts or fresh berries.

A Meditation to Release Attachments

Sit comfortably with your spine straight and your eyes closed. Take a few deep breaths and bring your focus inside your body. Now, envision the person or situation that you are currently attached to. See a long, thick rope all the way from your heart, wrapping around the person or situation. Next, welcome in an angel or a friend and watch as they take a giant pair of scissors and cut the rope between you and your attachment. See the rope fall, your end no longer attached as it crumbles into dust.

Take a deep breath in and feel the energetic release. See your former attachment through love and newfound freedom. Take a deep breath in and hold it, locking in this feeling of relief, and then exhale and relax. Repeat as often as necessary.

"

I surrender my attachments.

Chocolate "Caramel" Truffles

When you crave indulgent treats, tune into your body. Often, it's really asking for love, rest, and nutrition. Once you've given your body some divine self-care, you can responsibly enjoy a food treat out of love! These little truffles are a healthy version of a decadent treat that you can whip up in minutes.

YIELD: 12 truffles

13-ounce (375 g) package pitted dates
3 tablespoons (48 g) cashew butter
12-ounce (336 g) bag vegan sugar-free chocolate chips
2 tablespoons (24 g) raw extra-virgin coconut oil
Unsweetened coconut flakes or finely chopped cashews, for coating (optional)

Divine Bath-Time Relaxation

Draw a nice, hot bath filled with Epsom salts or bubbles. Light a few candles and play some soft, peaceful music. Pour yourself a big glass of water with lemon or cucumber. Sink into the bathwater, relaxing your entire body. Place one hand over your heart and one hand just below your navel point. Close your eyes and focus on your third-eye point. Take deep breaths in which your hands feel your body rising and falling. Hold the mantra, ***I am divine*** in your mind and repeat it silently, allowing it to clear your thoughts and ground you back in your truth. Continue doing this for the next 11 to 22 minutes, allowing yourself to be relaxed and held while you connect inward.

Line a baking sheet with parchment paper and set aside.

Combine the dates and cashew butter in a food processor and pulse until entirely clumped together. Transfer the mixture to a large bowl, scoop up a spoonful of mixture, and roll it into a 1-inch (2.5 cm) ball. Place the ball onto the prepared baking sheet, and then repeat until all the mixture is used. Freeze for 15 to 20 minutes.

Meanwhile, prepare the chocolate: Fill a medium saucepan half full with water and bring to a boil. Place the chocolate chips and coconut oil in a separate smaller saucepan, place the pan in the hot water, and heat, stirring continuously for 3 to 5 minutes, or until the chocolate has melted.

Remove the balls from the freezer. Using a toothpick, one by one dip the balls in the melted chocolate and then place them back onto the parchment paper. Put the coconut flakes or crushed cashews, if using, in a shallow bowl, coat the truffles, and place them back on the baking tray. Freezer for another 20 minutes, and then place in the refrigerator until ready to serve.

"

I treat myself divinely.

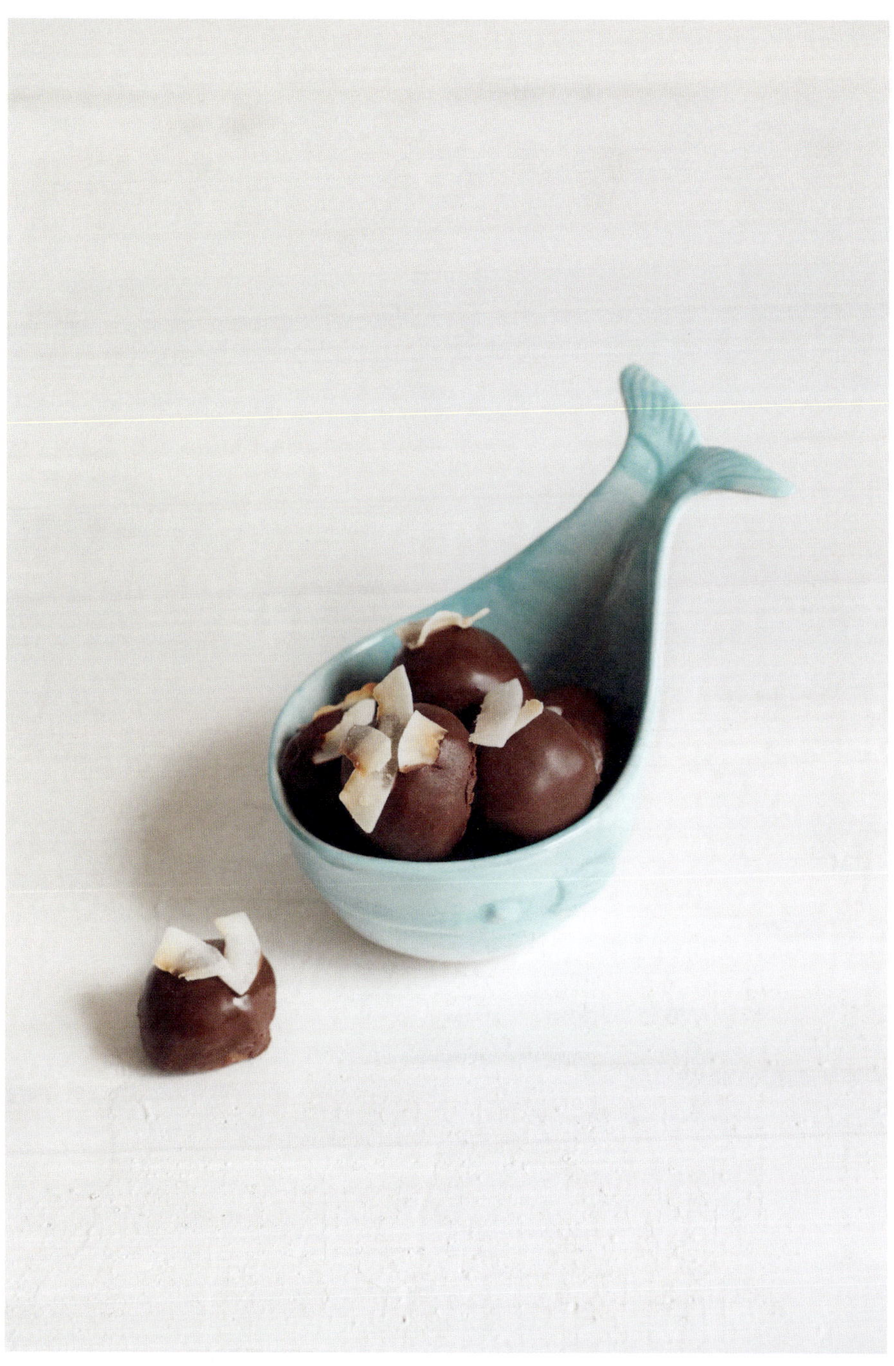

Mini Cheesecakes

Our bodies and souls crave adventure and variety—when we get stuck in a monotonous routine, we can start feeling depressed. I create adventure in my life in the kitchen! These cheesecakes were a product of that desire. I was tempted to make something for dessert that I had never made before.

YIELD: 12 mini cakes

CRUST
1 cup (175 g) pitted dates
3 tablespoons (19 g) chopped almonds
3 tablespoons (19 g) chopped walnuts
3 tablespoons (19 g) chopped hazelnuts
1 tablespoon (9 g) chia seeds
1 tablespoon (5 g) unsweetened cocoa powder
2 teaspoons vanilla extract
½ teaspoon ground cardamom

FILLING
1½ cups (195 g) raw unsalted cashew nuts, soaked in water for 2 to 3 hours and drained
Juice of 1 lemon
⅓ cup (66 g) raw extra-virgin coconut oil
½ cup (119 ml) canned coconut milk
1 tablespoon (15 ml) vanilla extract
2 teaspoons almond extract

GARNISH (OPTIONAL)
Raspberries
Unsweetened fruit jam
Cacao nibs
Almond butter

Line a 12-cup muffin pan with paper baking cups. To make the crust, combine all the ingredients in a food processor and pulse until well blended and clumpy. Roll a small amount of the mixture into a 2-inch (5 cm) ball and flatten it against the bottom of a muffin cup to form the crust for a cheesecake. Repeat with the remaining mixture, and then place the tray in the freezer.

Meanwhile, make the filling. Clean the food processor, add the filling ingredients, and purée until thick and creamy.

Remove the pan from the freezer and pour the filling evenly into each cup, until each is about full. If desired, add a few raspberries or, alternatively, top with a dollop of almond butter and a few cacao nibs.

Freeze for another 30 minutes, and then chill in the refrigerator until ready to serve!

“

 I make space for adventure.

Mystical Adventure Visualization

Find a comfortable spot where you can relax. Close your eyes and focus on your third-eye point. Take long, deep breaths, inhaling through your nose, deep into your diaphragm, and exhaling out your mouth. Bring to mind a place you would love to visit—whatever first comes to mind for you is perfect. Spend the next 11 minutes allowing yourself to explore that environment; wander around and have an experience. Allow any images that come up to be perfect and surrender to the journey. To end the meditation, take a deep breath in, come back to the room, then exhale. Rub your arms and legs with your hands to bring you back to Earth.

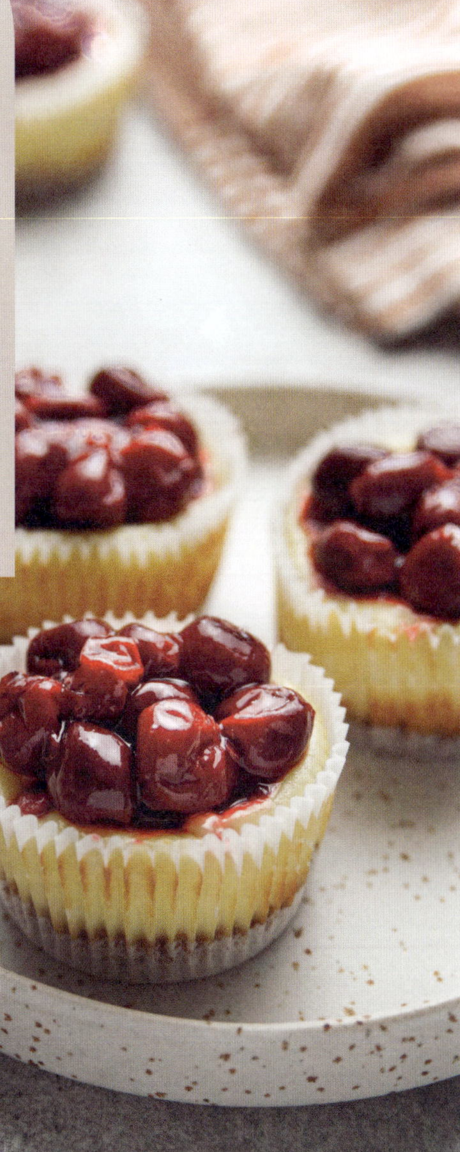

04

Winter

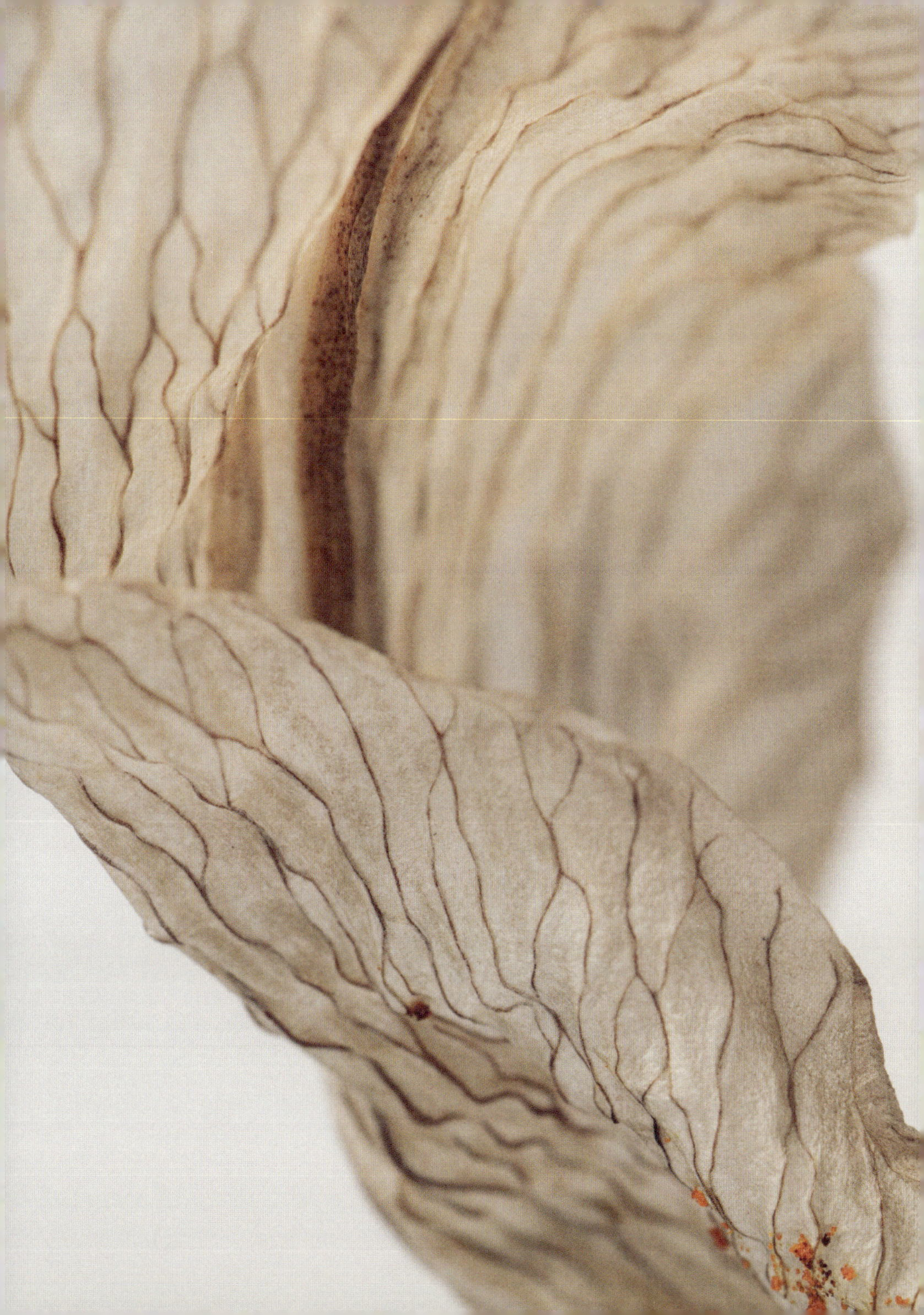

Deep-Healing Juice

This powerful tonic is my secret to getting back on my feet in no time when I'm feeling under the weather. Along with the usual healing suspects, such as ginger and turmeric, I've added my secret weapon: oregano oil. It pairs wonderfully with the healing meditation below.

YIELD: 1 serving

3 oranges, peeled and quartered
1 grapefruit, peeled and quartered
2-inch (5 cm) piece ginger root
2-inch (5 cm) piece turmeric root
2 to 4 drops oregano essential oil (this oil can be potent, so I recommend starting out with a small amount)

Juice all the ingredients except the oregano oil into a large glass.

Add the oregano oil, stir well, and serve immediately.

Healing Light Meditation

You may want to take a short nap following this meditation and let it all soak in.

Cover a bed, couch, or yoga mat with a soft blanket and lie down on your back. Close your eyes and turn your focus to your breath, breathing in deeply through your nose and out your mouth. Allow your breath to circulate throughout your body, feeling it in every nook and cranny and clearing it out on your exhale, releasing toxins out of your body. Repeat this for several breaths and then visualize a bright green light and welcome it in. Feel this light penetrate every part of your body, especially those areas that need healing—envision it infiltrating every cell in those areas and restoring them to health. When you are ready, take a deep breath in and hold it, allowing the green light to flood your entire system and soak up any toxic impurities, then exhale powerfully and release them out of your system.

"

I am well.

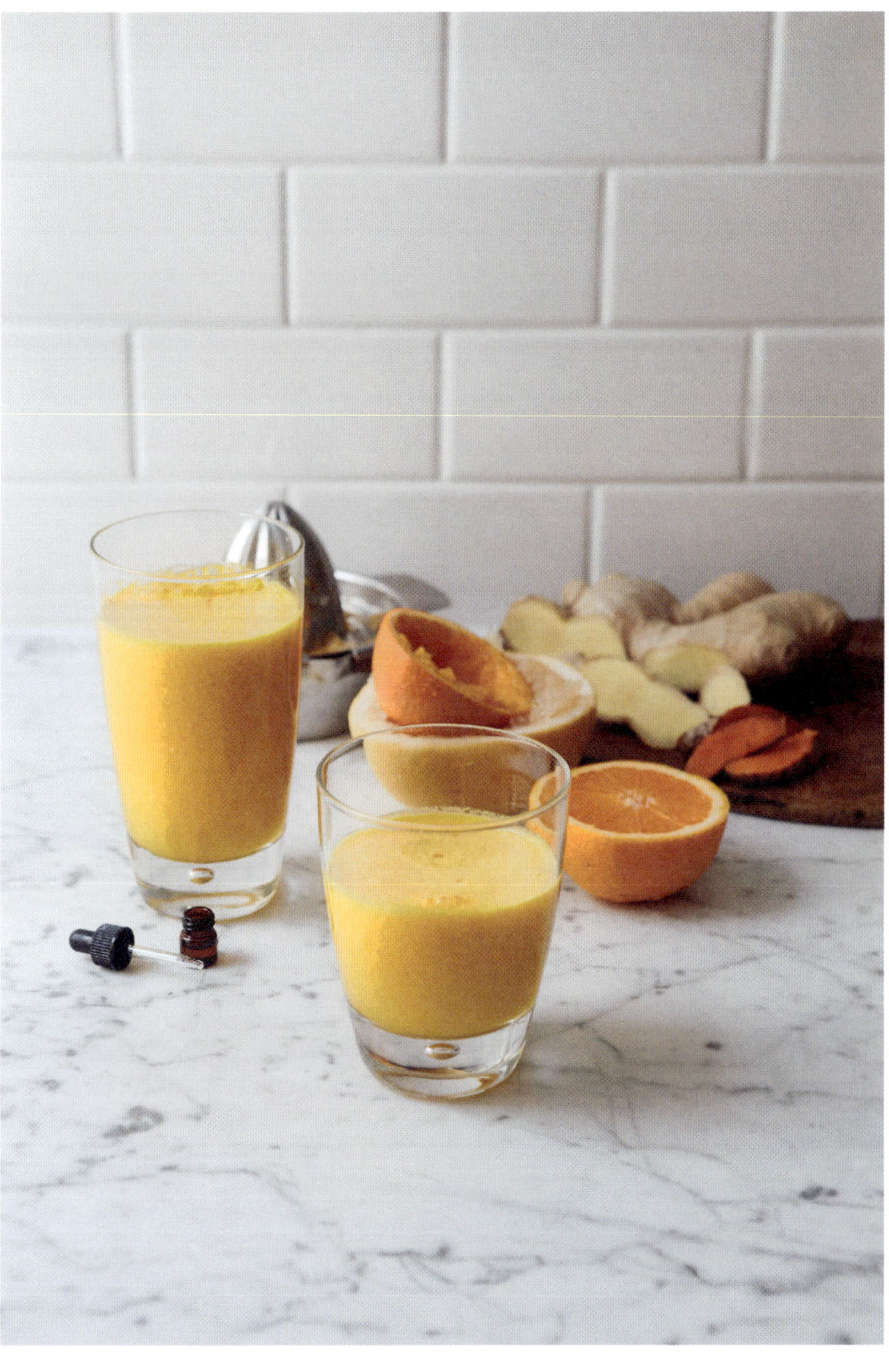

Standard Green Machine

The activating Kundalini meditation below helps energize your system and clear your head—a potent one-two punch when combined with a morning green juice like this one, loaded with alkalizing vegetables to help cure that brain fog and give you a boost to get through your day!

YIELD: 1 serving

3 celery stalks
1 green apple, coarsely chopped
½ cucumber, peeled
½ lemon, peeled
3 cups (90 g) spinach
2 cups (134 g) chopped kale
2-inch (5 cm) piece ginger root

Juice all the ingredients into a large glass. Lightly stir and serve immediately.

Ego Eradicator

Sit cross-legged with your hands in prayer position at your heart's center. Tune in with the adi mantra

ong-namo-guru-dev-namo

three times. Then raise your arms to 60 degrees, touch your fingers to the pads of your palms (as if you're filing your nails) and stick your thumbs up like you are plugging them into the ceiling). Now begin sharply exhaling and inhaling through your nose, focusing on the exhale (imagine blowing out a candle with your nose, then allow the inhale to naturally match it). Keep this breath going for 1 minute at first, gradually building up to 11 minutes. When time is up, take a deep breath and keep your hands up, allowing your thumbs to move toward each other until they are touching. Release your fingers and exhale after 10 seconds. Allow your hands to float down to the sides of your body and touch the floor. Sit and enjoy the crystal-clear energy flowing throughout your system.

“

I choose to fuel myself with pure, clean energy.

Avocado Black Bean Hash

Often when we reach for more filling comfort foods, it's because we don't feel full within ourselves. A nice hearty breakfast gives me the energy to move through my day feeling grounded and supported in my body, and this hash can be thrown together quickly.

YIELD: 2 to 4 servings

3 tablespoons (45 ml) extra-virgin olive oil, divided
6 small fingerling (or new) potatoes, sliced into ¼-inch-thick (6 mm) rounds
Salt and freshly ground black pepper, to taste
1 red onion, diced
2 avocados, halved and pitted, divided
1 green pepper, seeded and chopped
1 cup (172 g) precooked black beans, drained and rinsed
1 cup (150 g) cherry tomatoes, halved
½ cup (82 g) corn kernels

Preheat the oven to 425°F (220°C, or gas mark 7). Use 1 tablespoon (15 ml) olive oil to lightly grease a medium baking sheet. Spread out the potatoes and lightly season with salt and pepper. Roast in the oven for 5 minutes, or until the edges start to brown.

In the meantime, heat the remaining 2 tablespoons (30 ml) oil in a large frying pan over medium heat. Sauté the onion for 3 to 4 minutes, or until it starts to brown. Chop one of the avocados, stir it into the pan, and then add the green pepper, black beans, tomatoes, and corn. Reduce the heat to low. Add the potatoes to the pan and increase the heat to medium.

Mix for another 1 to 2 minutes, and then transfer to a serving dish. Slice the remaining avocado, add to the dish, and serve.

PUMP UP THE PROTEIN:
Simply add the tofu scramble from the Brunch Tacos recipe (page 39) to get some additional protein into this meal.

Light-Filled Meditation

Sit cross-legged with your palms facing up. Start taking long, deep breaths in through your nose and out your mouth. Visualize a golden ball of divine light at the center of your being, and with each inhale, see that golden light expand and grow brighter. Keep breathing as the light expands to fill up your entire being. Allow the light to expand beyond your body and surround you in a golden ball. Take this energy in, and feel how you are supported and held from your own inner light source. Continue for 3 minutes, then take a deep breath in, hold it, and allow the golden light to saturate every cell of your being. Exhale and relax.

"

I am full within myself.

Cherry Rosemary Scones

Do you have parts that you smooth over for others? What would happen if you embraced them instead? Playing around with different flavor combinations for these scones, I found the cherry-rosemary pairing to be delightfully surprising, quirky, and well-balanced—they're not too sweet and just a little savory.

YIELD: 8 to 10 scones

⅓ cup (66 g) melted raw extra-virgin coconut oil, plus 1 teaspoon for greasing
2 cups (296 g) gluten-free 1-to-1 flour
3 tablespoons (29 g) date sugar (coconut or maple sugar work as well)
1 tablespoon (15 ml) baking powder
Pinch of salt
1 cup (238 g) canned full-fat coconut milk
2 teaspoons vanilla extract
3 tablespoons (5 g) finely chopped fresh rosemary
1 cup (154 g) pitted cherries, halved

Preheat the oven to 375°F (190°C, or gas mark 5) and grease a small baking sheet (or a scone pan) with 1 teaspoon coconut oil.

In a medium mixing bowl, combine all the dry ingredients and mix thoroughly, breaking up any clumps. Add the melted coconut oil, coconut milk, vanilla extract, and chopped rosemary, mix thoroughly, and then gently fold in the cherries. (The batter should be thick like cookie dough.)

Roll the batter into a ball, place it on the greased baking sheet, and press down to make a 2-inch (5 cm) thick disk. Bake for 11 to 13 minutes, or until the edges crisp and a fork comes out clean when inserted into the center. Set aside to cool for 15 minutes, and then use a sharp knife or pizza cutter to slice into 8 to 10 slices. (Alternatively, cut batter into rounds and bake.)

GET CREATIVE:
While I do find the cherry-rosemary combo fabulous, there are many easy ways to switch up the flavor of these scones. Some of my favorite combos are blueberry-basil, strawberry-chocolate chips, scallion-garlic, and plant-based smoked gouda-caramelized onions. Simply sub out the same quantities of the cherries and rosemary and voilà! Enjoy the unlimited possibilities!

"

I embrace my quirks with love.

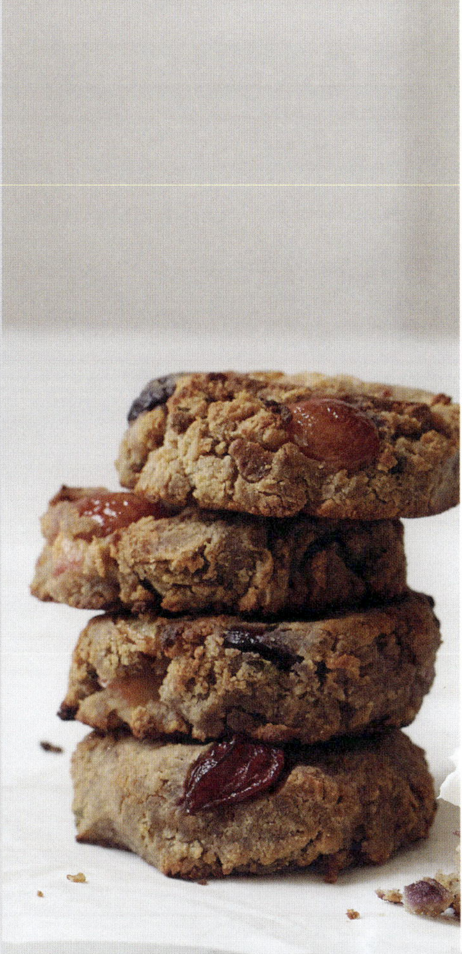

Unconditional Love Meditation

Close your eyes and sit down in easy pose. Start taking long, deep breaths, in through your nose and out through your mouth. Place one hand on your heart and the other hand over your navel, connecting with your body, your being, the very essence of who you are. Take a moment to see, feel, and acknowledge yourself as you would someone you deeply love like a romantic partner, close friend, or family member.

As you breathe and allow your awareness to drift inward, feel your hands holding your body with love. Spend the next 5 to 10 minutes looking at yourself and your body the way you would look at a loved one. Notice what shifts when you look through these eyes. Feel the love, acceptance, and grace that you so freely give to others return to you, reflected in your relationship with yourself. Sit in this feeling and let it saturate every cell of your being.

When you're ready, imagine a beautiful, loving light coming out of your hands and going into your body. Feel that love circulating as you give and receive love to yourself. Take a deep breath in and hold it, locking in this unconditional love. Exhale and open your eyes.

Flaxseed Pancakes

What fear has been holding you back? Your fear means well, but the life of your dreams is waiting for you on the other side of that fear. Pancakes are perfect for helping build intuition. You have to feel when a pancake is ready to be flipped. Sometimes it turns out messy and sometimes you time it perfectly, but it tastes delicious no matter how it looks.

YIELD: 3 pancakes

1 tablespoon (9 g) flaxseeds
3 (or 6, if using egg substitute) tablespoons (45 or 90 ml) water
1 tablespoon vegan egg substitute (optional for firmer consistency)
1 cup (227 g) coconut cream yogurt
½ cup (47 g) oat bran
2 teaspoons vanilla extract
½ teaspoon ground cinnamon (optional)
2 tablespoons (24 g) raw extra-virgin coconut oil, divided
1 cup (123 g) raspberries, to serve

To make flax "egg," mix the flaxseeds and 3 tablespoons water in a small bowl and set aside for 5 minutes, until thickened. If you'd like to use vegan egg substitute for a firmer consistency, mix your egg substitute powder with an additional 3 tablespoons of water and add the mixture to the bowl.

In a small mixing bowl, combine the flax "egg," yogurt, oat bran, vanilla extract, and cinnamon (if using), and mix well.

In a frying pan, heat 1 tablespoon (12 g) coconut oil over low heat. Scoop 2 tablespoons (30 g) of batter into the frying pan and cook, flipping over after 3 to 4 minutes or when the batter starts bubbling; cook for another 3 to 4 minutes. Transfer the pancake to a serving plate, and repeat with the remaining batter.

Clean the frying pan, and then heat the remaining tablespoon (12 g) coconut oil over medium-high heat. Add the raspberries to the pan and heat for 1 minute, until warmed through. The raspberries can be served on top or puréed to make a warm, sweet syrup!

GET CREATIVE:
These pancakes are also delicious with your favorite fruit added to them, like bananas or blueberries. Feel free to add some dairy-free chocolate chips or sprinkles to the mix to make them even more festive for a special occasion!

"

I am ready to take a leap of faith.

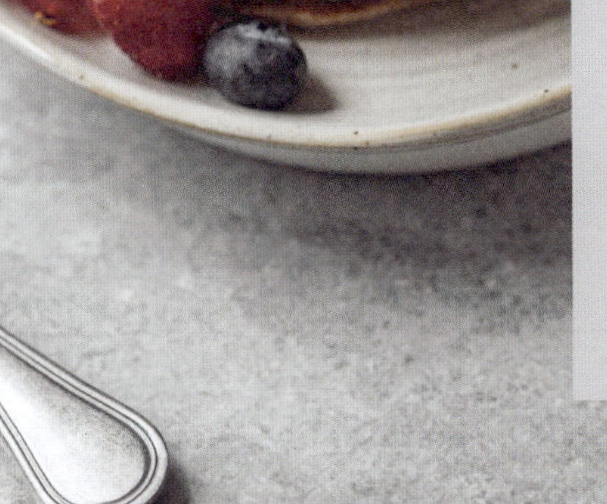

Tapping Through Your Fears

Sit in a chair with your feet placed firmly on the floor. Bring your left hand up in a karate chop gesture with the thumb towards your chest, tap the side of your left hand just below the pinkie with your right finger pads. (You can find an example of EFT tapping on my YouTube channel if it's hard to visualize. I have a playlist of videos with different themes and intentions.)

Continue tapping and speak the following aloud:

I am ready to release my fears, and I love and accept myself.

I am ready to release my fears, and I love and honor myself.

I am ready to release my fears, and I love and forgive myself.

Then continue speaking aloud about the specific fears that you are ready to release. Get it all out, allowing yourself to feel all the things these fears bring up as you continue tapping.

When you are feeling more peaceful, end your session with saying:

I release all these fears from my mind, body, and soul.

I release all these fears from my cells and my magnetic field.

I am ready to move forward without fear. I am excited to move forward without these fears.

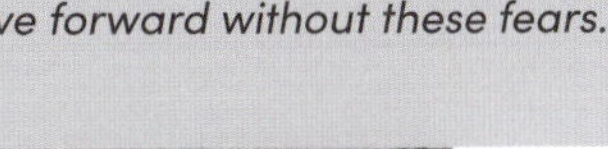

Strawberry-Banana "Hug" Cakes

Take the time today to sit in the feeling of love and support you have inside. These oatmeal cakes are my favorite winter breakfast and feel like a hug in your tummy. Freeze them to have on hand for a quick morning pick-me-up.

YIELD: 12 cakes

Coconut oil cooking spray, for greasing
2 teaspoons flaxseed meal
2 tablespoons (30 ml) water
3 cups (270 g) gluten-free quick oats
2 ripe bananas, mashed
½ cup (83 g) chopped strawberries
½ cup (122 g) unsweetened applesauce
¼ cup (60 ml) maple syrup
1 tablespoon (15 ml) baking powder
2 teaspoons ground cinnamon
2 teaspoons vanilla extract
½ teaspoon sea salt
Unsweetened almond or coconut milk, warmed, to serve (optional)
Fresh berries, to garnish (optional)

Preheat the oven to 375°F (190°C, or gas mark 5). Grease a 12-cup muffin pan with cooking spray.

To make flax "egg," mix together the flaxseed and water in a small bowl and set aside for 5 minutes, until thickened.

In a medium mixing bowl, combine the flax "egg," oats, bananas, strawberries, applesauce, maple syrup, baking powder, ground cinnamon, vanilla extract, and sea salt, and gently mix. Scoop the mixture into the prepared muffin pan until two-thirds full and bake for 7 to 10 minutes, or until a light crust forms on top. Remove and set aside to cool.

Serve as is or place the baked oatmeal in a bowl of warm almond or coconut milk and garnish with fresh berries.

Meditation for a Broken Heart

This deceptively simple meditation calms the mind and body, allowing your nervous system to move out of fight-or-flight and back into a serene space of love and safety. Sit cross-legged and wrap your arms around yourself in a firm embrace. Close your eyes and begin taking deep breaths. Feel your arms holding you. Allow this physical sensation of being held to permeate your being, receiving the peace and calm it brings you. Allow the part of you that is hurting to arise within and speak to you about what it's experiencing as you continue to firmly hold the embrace, giving comfort to this vulnerable part of yourself. Continue as long as needed. End your meditation with a deep breath in, holding it for a count of 10 and then exhaling powerfully as you open your eyes.

"

I am loved and supported.

Mushroom Barley Soup

Dig down deep into that inner well of strength and you will always persevere. The healing energy of mushrooms and the good-for-your-gut barley in this hearty soup will help build that strength!

YIELD: 4 servings

3 tablespoons (45 ml) extra-virgin olive oil
½ white onion, diced
1 clove garlic, chopped
1 cup (70 g) sliced cremini mushrooms
1 package (3.5 ounces/85 g) enoki mushrooms
1 maitake (hen of the woods) mushroom, chopped
4 cups (960 ml) mushroom broth
1 cup (157 g) cooked barley (or gluten-free quinoa)
2 cups (136 g) chopped kale or spinach
2 tablespoons (30 ml) onion powder
1½ tablespoons (23 g) fresh thyme leaves
1 tablespoon (15 ml) salt, plus extra to taste

Heat the olive oil in a large frying pan over medium heat. Add the onions and sauté for 5 minutes until softened, then add the garlic and sauté for another minute. Stir in the mushrooms and sauté for another 2 to 3 minutes, until the mushrooms are browned.

Pour in the mushroom broth, add the barley (or quinoa), kale, onion powder, thyme, and salt, and stir. Bring to a boil, then reduce the heat, and simmer for 10 minutes. Season with more salt to taste.

Meditation for Filling Up Your Well

Sit cross-legged with your hands facing palms up on your knees. Start taking long, deep breaths and connect internally with how you are feeling in this moment. After a couple minutes, visualize an "energy tank" of sorts around your navel center. How much light fuel do you currently see in your tank? Observe it without judgment, simply noting the level. Then, visualize two tubes connecting to that energy tank, one going up to the heavens and the other going down into the Earth. Open the flow to receive more fuel for your tank, envisioning white light flowing down from the heavens into your well, while simultaneously watching the deep golden light coming up from the core of the Earth. Let these flows mix together in your energy tank.

Stay here until your tank is full. When you are done, thank both sources for the renewed energy, and allow the tubes to retreat into your well. Open your eyes and go enjoy your new reserves of fuel!

"

I have the strength to persevere.

Interconnectedness Meditation

Get outside if possible: go to a park, the beach, or someplace where you feel peaceful and connected to the Earth. Sit comfortably with your spine straight and your eyes closed. Rest your palms face up on your knees. Take a deep breath in through your nose and out your mouth. Take a few long, deep breaths, allowing any tension or stress from the day to release from your body. Bring your focus to your sitting bones; feel them supporting you. Imagine a root growing out of your spine and reaching all the way to the core of the Earth and anchoring you. Feel it supporting you and holding you. Now bring your focus to the top of your head. Feel a warm, white light pouring down from above and coming in through the crown of your head, filling your body with its warmth and light. Allow yourself to sit in this space, being held from both directions, filled with light and anchored to the Earth. When you are ready, take a deep breath in and hold it, filling yourself with this feeling Exhale and relax.

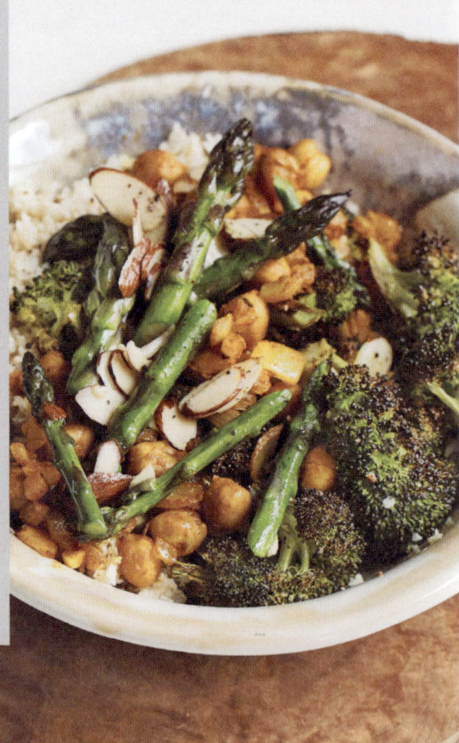

The Rooted Bowl

There is no greater power than realizing we are all one. Just as you are one person in the world, you are the world in one person. Eating this bowl filled with lots of roasted root veggies reconnects me to the earth and helps me feel strong and focused.

YIELD: 2 servings

Coconut oil cooking spray, for greasing
1 cup (100 g) cauliflower florets
1 cup (100 g) broccoli florets
Salt and freshly ground black pepper, to taste
2 tablespoons (30 ml) extra-virgin olive oil, divided
1 bunch asparagus spears, trimmed
2 cloves garlic, finely chopped
3 tablespoons (13 g) sliced almonds
1 small white onion, diced
2 teaspoons ground turmeric
2 teaspoons ground coriander
2 teaspoons curry powder
½ teaspoon paprika
15-ounce (425 g) can chickpeas, rinsed and drained

Preheat the oven to 425°F (220°C, or gas mark 7). Lightly grease 1 large or 2 medium baking sheets with the cooking spray.

Spread out your cauliflower and broccoli on the baking sheet(s). Lightly season with salt and pepper each and roast for 15 minutes.

Meanwhile, heat 1 tablespoon (15 ml) olive oil in a frying pan over medium heat. Add the asparagus and cook for 3 to 4 minutes, until they turn bright green. Add the garlic and almonds and sauté for another minute. Transfer the asparagus to a bowl.

Using the same frying pan, heat the remaining 1 tablespoon (15 ml) olive oil over medium heat. Add the onion, turmeric, coriander, curry, and paprika and cook for 2 to 3 minutes. Stir in the chickpeas, mix well so that they are covered in the spices, and cook for another 5 minutes. Set aside.

Remove the roasted broccoli and cauliflower from the oven and put them into individual serving bowls. (Alternatively, put the cauliflower in a food processor and pulse a few times until it has a rice-like consistency, as shown in the photograph. Then place the rice and broccoli in your bowls.)

To serve, scatter over the chickpeas and top with the asparagus.

“

I am connected to everything.

Yogi Bowl

I'm a huge lover of the "yogi bowl." It gives you permission to put together a few of your favorite things and call it a meal. It's great for leftovers and for making healthy choices when you are short on time—it will fill you up so you can shine bright all day long.

YIELD: 2 servings

OPTION 1

1 cup (185 g) cooked quinoa
1 avocado, halved, pitted, and diced
2 cups (272 g) steamed veggies such as broccoli, cauliflower, or zucchini (you can use fresh, frozen, or a steam-bag option)
1 cup (185 g) precooked black beans, rinsed, drained, and warmed

DIJON VINAIGRETTE

¼ cup (60 ml) extra-virgin olive oil
¼ cup (60 g) Dijon mustard
2 tablespoons (30 ml) balsamic vinegar
2 tablespoons (20 g) freshly grated horseradish
Salt and freshly ground black pepper, to taste
Grade B maple syrup (optional, for a maple-Dijon dressing), to taste

To make my favorite Dijon vinaigrette, combine all the ingredients in a small bowl and whisk until creamy.

Combine all the other ingredients in a bowl, drizzle over the dressing, and toss. Serve. (Alternatively, serve the dressing on the side.)

GET CREATIVE:

Feel free to exchange the black beans for another source of protein, like tempeh or tofu.

Kundalini Mantra for Self-Esteem

You can choose to do this exercise as a standard meditation or a living meditation. For the standard version, sit comfortably, close your eyes, and focus on your third-eye point (the space between your eyebrows), and repeat:

I am bountiful, blissful, and beautiful. Bountiful, blissful, and beautiful, I am.

There are also great recordings on YouTube or Spotify that you can sing along with if that is your thing. Continue for anywhere from 3 to 11 minutes and then take a deep breath in, hold it, and exhale.

As a living meditation, bring the mantra with you wherever you go, repeating it silently in your head.

It's a great counterbalance to negative self-talk. When you hear your mean inner voice come up, bring up the mantra and replace any nonloving thoughts with this simple self-affirming phrase.

"

I am bountiful, blissful, and beautiful.

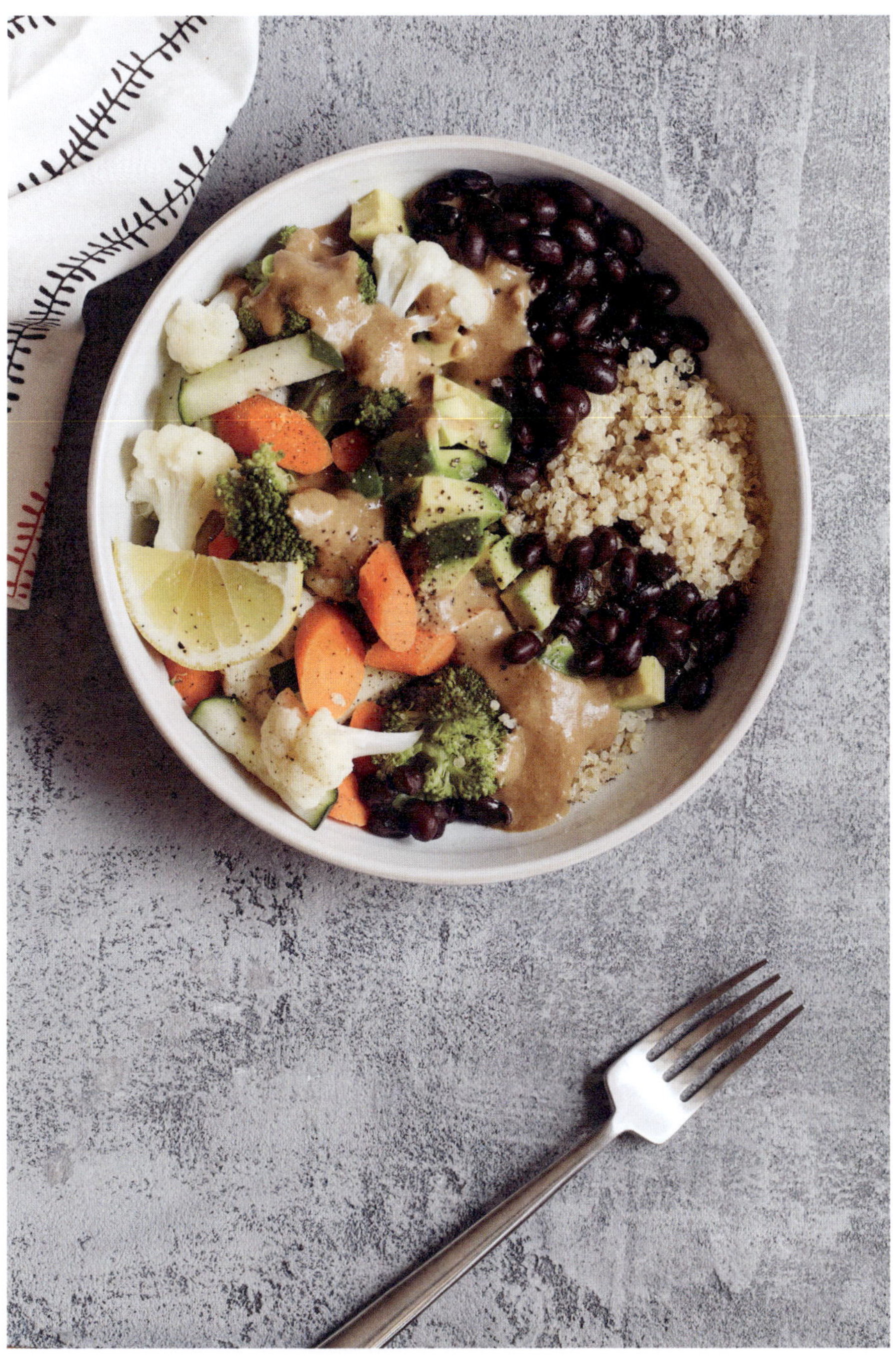

Grandma's Galumpkis (Stuffed Cabbage Rolls)

I lost my grandma in January of 2021, and her passing left such a hole in my heart. I miss her wise words and loving advice deeply. This is a recreated a dish from my grandma's childhood. She used to love these galumpkis when she was growing up. They are normally filled with rice and chopped meat, but this plant-based version calls for filling them with vegetables, lentils, and rice.

YIELD: 4 servings

Coconut oil cooking spray, for greasing
2 Japanese eggplants, halved

SAUCE
2 tablespoons (30 ml) extra-virgin olive oil
1 clove garlic, finely chopped
(2) 28-ounce (794 g) cans crushed tomatoes
2 tablespoons (30 ml) apple cider vinegar
2 teaspoons onion powder
2 teaspoons oregano
2 teaspoons basil
½ teaspoon salt
½ teaspoon pepper

FILLING
2 tablespoons (30 ml) extra-virgin olive oil
1 yellow onion, diced
1 clove garlic, finely chopped
2 tablespoons (8 g) finely chopped fresh parsley
2 tablespoons (32 g) tomato paste
2 cups (400 g) cooked green lentils
1½ cups (293 g) cooked brown rice
Salt and freshly ground black pepper, to taste
2 large heads green cabbage, halved and core removed

Meditation for Connecting to a Departed Loved One

This is a simple practice to help you connect with and receive guidance from a loved one who is no longer with you. Sit or lie down and completely relax with your eyes closed. Take a few deep breaths and bring your awareness to your heart center. Call up an image of your missing loved one. See their smiling face and breathe in their loving presence. You may want to spend a few minutes simply sitting here, enjoying this. When you are ready, ask them your question and allow yourself to receive the guidance they have for you. Be patient with yourself if this is a new practice for you. Surrender to their loving image in your mind and trust what arises. When you are ready, thank them and tell them anything else you want to share before closing the meditation and bringing yourself back to the present moment. Go forth knowing that they are always right there in your heart.

Preheat the oven to 375°F (190°C, or gas mark 5). Lightly grease a medium baking sheet with cooking spray.

Slice the eggplants vertically and then lay the slices between layers of paper towels to draw out moisture. Place the eggplants on the prepared baking sheet and roast for 15 minutes, or until they begin to brown. Set aside but leave the oven on (to bake the cabbage rolls).

To make the sauce, heat the olive oil in a large saucepan over medium heat, add the garlic, and sauté for 1 to 2 minutes. Add the crushed tomatoes, apple cider vinegar, onion powder, oregano, basil, salt, and pepper. Bring to a boil, reduce the heat, and simmer for 5 minutes. Set aside.

To make the filling, heat the olive oil in another large saucepan over medium heat. Add the onions and sauté for 5 minutes, until softened, then add the garlic and sauté for another minute. Add the roasted eggplant, parsley, tomato paste, ½ cup (125 g) sauce, lentils, and brown rice and mix until thoroughly combined. Season with salt and pepper to taste. Remove from the heat and transfer the mixture to a bowl.

Fill a small bowl with cold water and set aside. Fill a large saucepan halfway with water and bring to a boil over high heat. Gently pull apart each leaf of cabbage, blanch in the boiling water for 1 to 2 minutes or until pliable, and then use a slotted spoon to transfer the cabbage leaves into the bowl of cold water.

Line the bottom of a 9 x 13-inch (23 x 33 cm) baking dish (or two 9-inch, or 23 cm, round pans) with broken or l ess-attractive leaves until entirely covered. Put a cabbage leaf on a clean work surface and place a teaspoon to a tablespoon of filling in the center of the leaf. Roll up the leaf, tucking the sides in, to create a little package. Place the roll, seam side down, in your dish. Continue with the remaining leaves and filling.

Pour the remaining sauce over the rolls and bake for 30 minutes, or until the leaves lining the dish begin to brown. Serve.

“

I handle all situations with grace and courage.

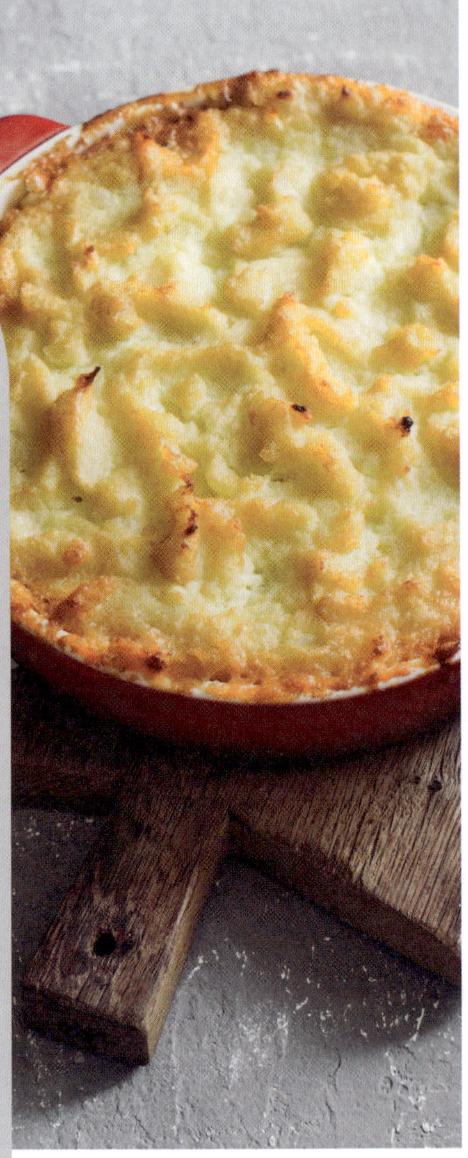

Butterfly Recalibration Meditation

This meditation helps shift your nervous system from fight-or-flight mode to feeling safe, peaceful, and trusting in the divine unfolding of your life.

Sit in a chair with both feet on the floor and your arms crossed over your chest, palms against the front of the opposite arm. Close your eyes and bring to mind a situation in your life right now where you are feeling impatient, frustrated, or disappointed. Allow yourself to notice where these feelings live in your body. Begin tapping or "butterflying" the palms of your hands one at time, alternating "wing flaps" of each hand, as you allow yourself to breathe through the feelings, thoughts, and images arising in your body and mind. Continue for 3 to 5 minutes or until you start feeling more relaxed, while holding this situation in your consciousness. Silently repeat this affirmation:

Everything in my life is happening for me. It is all leading me to my greatest desires. I am safe to trust the process.

Repeat this in your head while simultaneously holding the situation until it feels true in your body. Open your eyes and shake out your hands to close.

Lentil Shepherd's Pie

Who doesn't love a nice hearty dish, especially in the winter, that makes you feel like you are wrapped in a blanket? I like making this dish for friends on a Sunday and eating the leftovers all week for lunch.

YIELD: 8 servings

FILLING
2 tablespoons (30 ml) extra-virgin olive oil
1 white onion, diced
1 clove garlic
1½ cups (264 g) dried green lentils
4 cups (960 ml) mushroom stock
3 sprigs of rosemary, plus extra to garnish
Coconut oil cooking spray, for greasing
½ cup (61 g) thinly sliced and halved carrots
½ cup (73 g) peas
½ cup (34 g) baby kale
¼ cup (41 g) corn kernels
2 tablespoons (30 ml) arrowroot powder (optional)
Salt, to taste

TOPPING
5 Yukon gold potatoes, peeled and sliced
Salt, to taste
2 tablespoons (30 ml) extra-virgin olive oil
1 white onion, diced
1 clove garlic, chopped
¼ cup (56 g) vegan butter
¼ cup (60 g) unsweetened almond milk
Freshly ground black pepper, to taste

To make the filling, heat the oil in a large frying pan over medium heat. Add the onions and sauté for 5 minutes until softened, then add the garlic and sauté for another minute. Add the lentils, mushroom stock, and rosemary. Bring to a gentle boil, then reduce the heat and simmer for 35 minutes.

To make the topping, put the potatoes in a large saucepan, cover with water, and add salt. Bring to a gentle boil over medium-high heat, and then cover and cook for 20 minutes, or until the potatoes have softened. Drain and set aside.

Heat the oil in a frying pan over medium heat. Add the onion and sauté for 5 minutes, until softened, then add the garlic and sauté for another minute.

Transfer the potatoes, onion mixture, vegan butter, and almond milk to a blender or food processor. Pulse until just combined. Season with salt and pepper.

Meanwhile, preheat the oven to 425°F (220°C, or gas mark 7). Lightly grease a round, 2-quart (2 L) baking dish.

Add the carrots, peas, baby kale, and corn to the frying pan of lentils and cook for another 5 to 10 minutes, until the carrots are tender. Add the arrowroot powder to thicken the mixture, if desired. Remove the sprigs of rosemary, season with salt, and transfer the mixture to the baking dish.

Scoop the mashed potato topping over the lentil mixture until it's entirely covered. Bake in the oven for 10 to 15 minutes, or until the potatoes start to brown. Garnish with chopped rosemary and serve!

"

I feel loved and supported.

Spaghetti Squash with Fresh Herbs

It's time to pare down and let go of the white noise so that you can focus on what counts and get back in the flow. This dish is a wonderful example of how delicious things are just as they are. Fresh herbs are excellent for activating your clarity of mind, while the spaghetti squash is naturally grounding, allowing you to be both centered and clear at once.

YIELD: 2 servings

1 spaghetti squash
2 tablespoons (30 ml) extra-virgin olive oil, divided
1 bulb roasted garlic (see step 3 of Best Veggie Burger Ever and Avocado Fries, page 85), chopped
1 tablespoon (2 g) chopped fresh rosemary
1 tablespoon (2 g) chopped fresh oregano
1 tablespoon (2 g) chopped fresh thyme
1 tablespoon (2 g) chopped fresh basil
Juice of 1 lemon
½ teaspoon salt
½ cup shredded vegan parmesan (optional, for a creamier, richer dish)

Preheat the oven to 425°F (220°C, or gas mark 7).

Using a fork, poke holes in the squash, place on a baking sheet, and roast on the middle rack for 45 minutes. Set aside and when cool enough to handle, slice it in half lengthwise. Scoop out the seeds and discard. Use a fork to scrape out the "spaghetti" strings and transfer to a bowl.

Heat 1 tablespoon (15 ml) olive oil in a frying pan over medium heat, add the chopped garlic, and cook for a few minutes until browned. Stir in the "spaghetti" and cook for another 2 to 3 minutes, then add the fresh chopped herbs and lemon juice.

Drizzle in the remaining 1 tablespoon (15 ml) olive oil and season with the salt. Toss briefly, then transfer to a bowl and serve.

"

I receive clarity through simplicity.

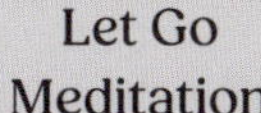

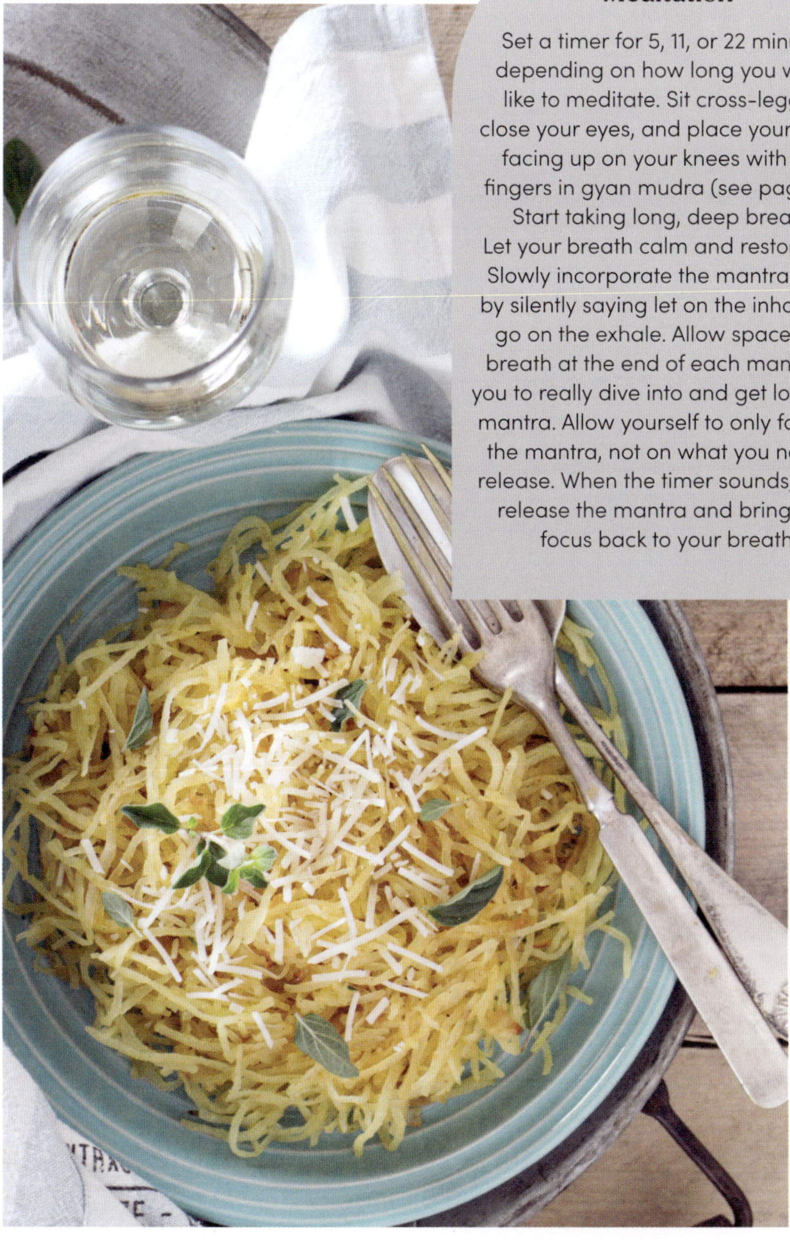

Let Go Meditation

Set a timer for 5, 11, or 22 minutes, depending on how long you would like to meditate. Sit cross-legged, close your eyes, and place your palms facing up on your knees with your fingers in gyan mudra (see page 68). Start taking long, deep breaths. Let your breath calm and restore you. Slowly incorporate the mantra let go by silently saying let on the inhale and go on the exhale. Allow space for a breath at the end of each mantra for you to really dive into and get lost in the mantra. Allow yourself to only focus on the mantra, not on what you need to release. When the timer sounds, gently release the mantra and bring your focus back to your breath.

Sweet Potato Pasta with Alfredo Sauce

When we are clear about what we truly desire, we open the door to unexpected opportunities. If you have been craving the warm, filling, creamy decadence of fettuccine Alfredo without the dairy and gluten, then this is the recipe for you. Talk about an unexpected way to get your cravings met!

YIELD: 2 servings

2 tablespoons (30 ml) extra-virgin olive oil
2 sweet potatoes, peeled and spiralized
Chopped walnuts, to garnish
Chopped parsley, to garnish

SAUCE
15-ounce (425 g) can cannellini beans, drained and rinsed
15-ounce (425 g) can chickpeas, drained and rinsed
½ cup (120 ml) unsweetened almond milk
7 tablespoons (105 g) nutritional yeast
3 tablespoons (45 ml) extra-virgin olive oil
2 tablespoons (30 g) Dijon mustard
1 tablespoon (14 g) vegan butter
1 tablespoon (15 ml) garlic powder
1 tablespoon (15 ml) salt, plus extra to taste
½ teaspoon ground turmeric

To make the sauce, combine all the sauce ingredients in a food processor and pulse until thick and creamy. Season with salt to taste.

Heat the olive oil in a medium saucepan and sauté the sweet potato "noodles" for 5 minutes, until softened. Add the sauce to the saucepan and cook for 2 to 3 minutes, until heated through. Garnish with the walnuts and parsley, and serve. (Alternatively, heat the sauce in a separate saucepan and ladle it over a plate of noodles.)

Feeling it Meditation

Sit cross-legged with your hands over your heart, eyes closed, breathing in through your nose and out your mouth. Allow yourself to fill up from your heart, radiating outward with the feelings of your desire fulfilled. Release any specific images that may come up and return to your heart and tune in to the feeling that is enveloping you around having what you truly desire. Sit in this feeling for the next 3 minutes. When time is up, take a deep breath in and silently say to yourself,

I release my attachment to what it looks like and I welcome in unexpected ways for it to manifest.

Exhale and relax.

"

I am open to unexpected opportunities.

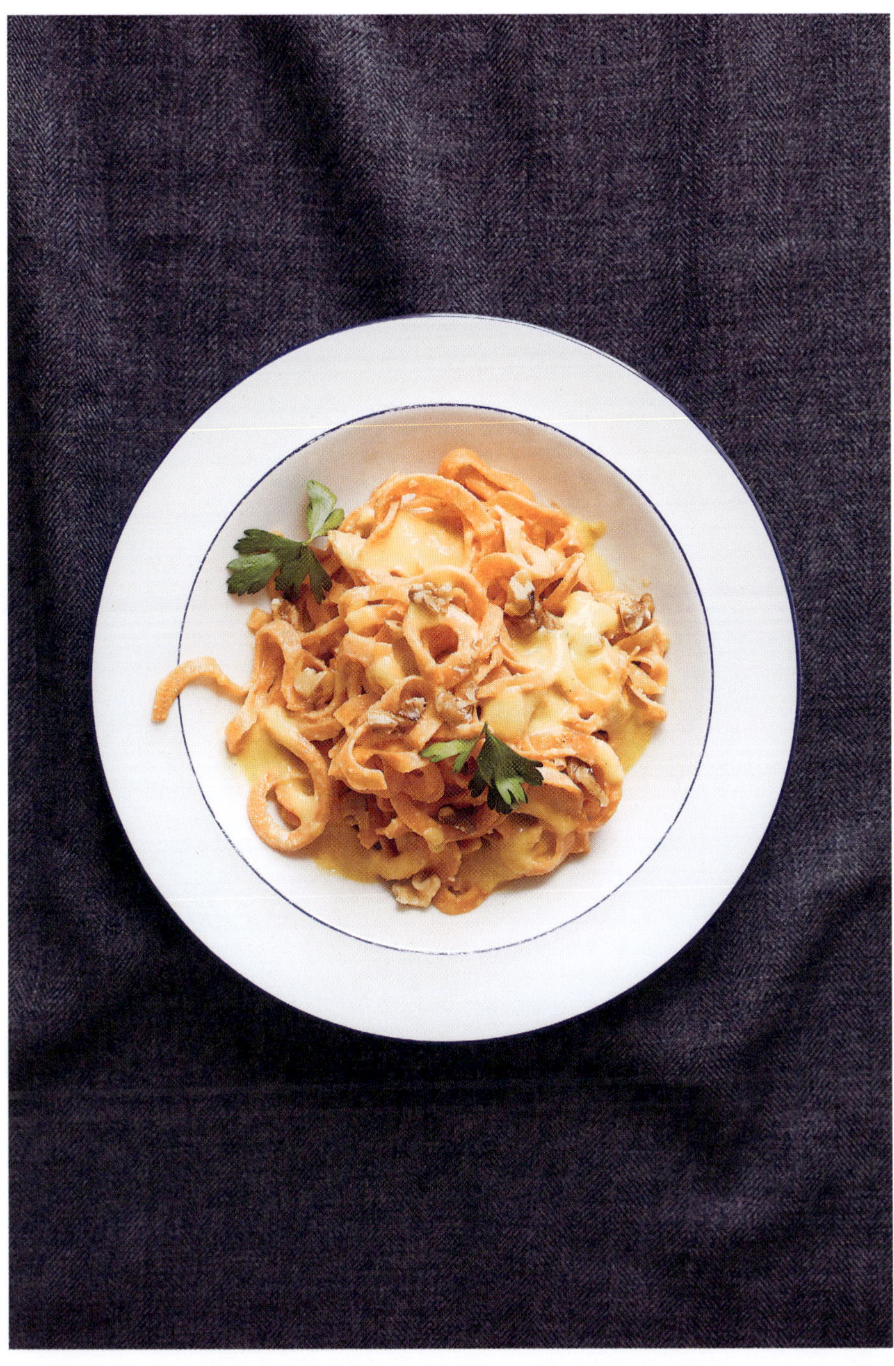

My Ideal Day Visualization

I invite you to blow the roof off what you think is possible for your life. Allow your mind to go where it wants and honor your deep desires, hopes, dreams, etc. You might even tap into dreams from your childhood. Have fun with it and you will gain some incredible insights. Find a comfortable spot to sit with your eyes closed and your palms facing up on your knees. Bring your focus inward, taking long, deep breaths, and imagine yourself waking up in the morning to your "ideal day." Visualize your bedroom, what does it look like? Take in the excitement you feel starting your day. Now, make your way through your day, observing as many details as possible: your morning routine, your outfit, your job, your dinner, and your nighttime routine. Take a moment to inhale deeply and hold it, allowing yourself to be filled with gratitude. Exhale. Slowly wiggle your hands and toes and come back into the room. If you like, jot down any details that you can start incorporating into your life right now.

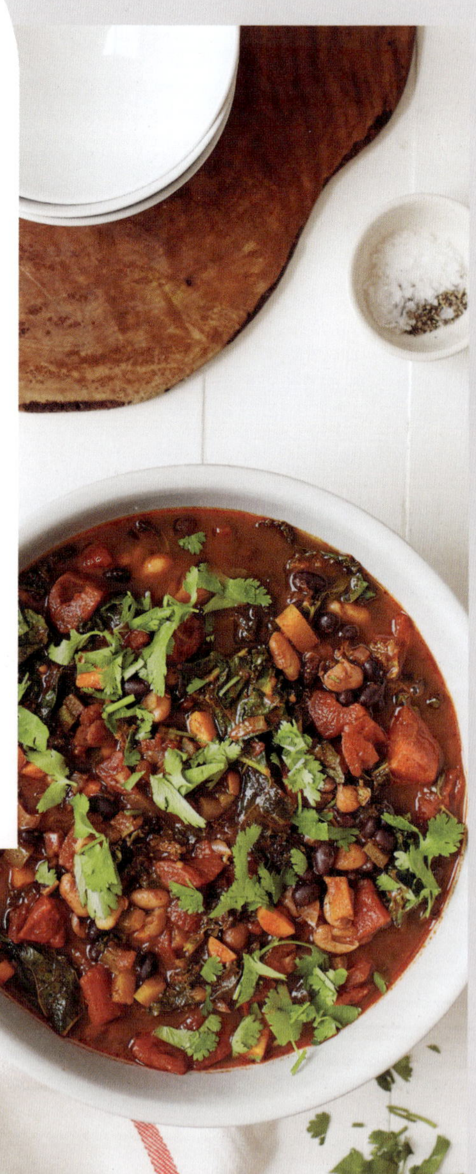

Veggie Chili

Just as you have the power to create your reality—through your thoughts, feelings, and subconscious patterns—with this chili, *you* decide what to put in and leave out.

YIELD: 4 servings

2 tablespoons (30 ml) extra-virgin olive oil
1 red onion, diced
4 garlic cloves, chopped
2 tablespoons (30 ml) chili powder
2 teaspoons ground cumin
1½ teaspoons smoked paprika
1 teaspoon dried oregano
2 carrots, chopped
1 large green pepper, seeded and chopped
28-ounce (800 g) can diced tomatoes
1 bay leaf
15-ounce (425 g) can black beans, rinsed and drained
15-ounce (425 g) can kidney beans rinsed and drained
2 cups (480 ml) vegetable broth
1 cup (140 g) chopped butternut squash
1 cup (68 g) chopped kale
1 to 2 teaspoons lime juice, to taste
Salt and freshly ground black pepper, to taste
2 tablespoons (2 g) chopped cilantro, to garnish

Heat the oil in a large saucepan over medium heat. Add the onions and sauté for 5 minutes until softened, then add the garlic and sauté for another minute. Stir in the chili powder, cumin, paprika, and oregano and cook for 1 to 2 minutes.

Add the remaining ingredients and bring to a boil over high heat. Reduce the heat and simmer for 15 to 20 minutes, stirring occasionally, until the carrots and squash are tender. Season with salt and pepper, transfer to serving bowls, and garnish with cilantro.

“

I am a powerful creator.

Chocolate Chip Hazelnut Heaven Cookies

When I first gave up dairy and gluten, I panicked thinking about life without chocolate chip cookies. It felt wrong and unfair, until one morning I got creative and made these delightful treats! This recipe reminds me that my inner critical voice is not me or my truth. With practice, I can choose to see the positive.

YIELD: 12 cookies

2 teaspoons flaxseed meal
2 tablespoons (30 ml) water
3 tablespoons (36 g) raw extra-virgin coconut oil, divided
1½ cups (141 g) gluten-free oat bran
2 tablespoons (32 g) cashew, almond, or hazelnut butter (I prefer the creamy sweetness of cashew butter)
1 large banana
½ cup (58 g) sliced hazelnuts
2 teaspoons vanilla extract
1 teaspoon almond extract
1 teaspoon ground cinnamon
½ cup (112 g) vegan sugar-free chocolate chips

Mix together the flaxseed meal and water in a bowl. Set aside for 5 minutes, until thickened.

Preheat the oven to 375°F (190°C, or gas mark 5) and grease a baking sheet with 1 tablespoon (12 g) coconut oil.

In a stand mixer, combine the oat bran, cashew butter, remaining 2 tablespoons (24 g) coconut oil, banana, hazelnuts, vanilla extract, almond extract, cinnamon, and flax "eggs." Mix on medium speed until thoroughly combined. Add the chocolate chips and mix on low speed. Using an ice-cream scooper or a tablespoon, scoop the cookie dough and place it on the baking sheet, about 2 inches (5 cm) apart. Bake for 10 to 12 minutes, or until the tops begin to dry.

Meditation for Self-Kindness

Sit cross-legged with your spine elongated and your eyes closed. Begin taking deep breaths in through your nose and out your mouth. Bring your focus to your heart center. Imagine a glowing ball of bright golden light in the center of your being. See it growing brighter with each breath. Now bring to mind the things you genuinely love about yourself. What endearing things do you do? Let your mind wander and allow it to flood you with all the beautiful facets of you—big and small. It's okay if you feel uncomfortable at first; we are not used to speaking to ourselves so sweetly, so it can feel a little strange. Relax, allow, and receive. Bask in your heart's expanding glow and continue for 3 minutes. Then take a deep breath in and hold it, infusing every cell of your body with that sweet, tender, loving-kindness. Exhale.

"

I speak sweetly to myself.

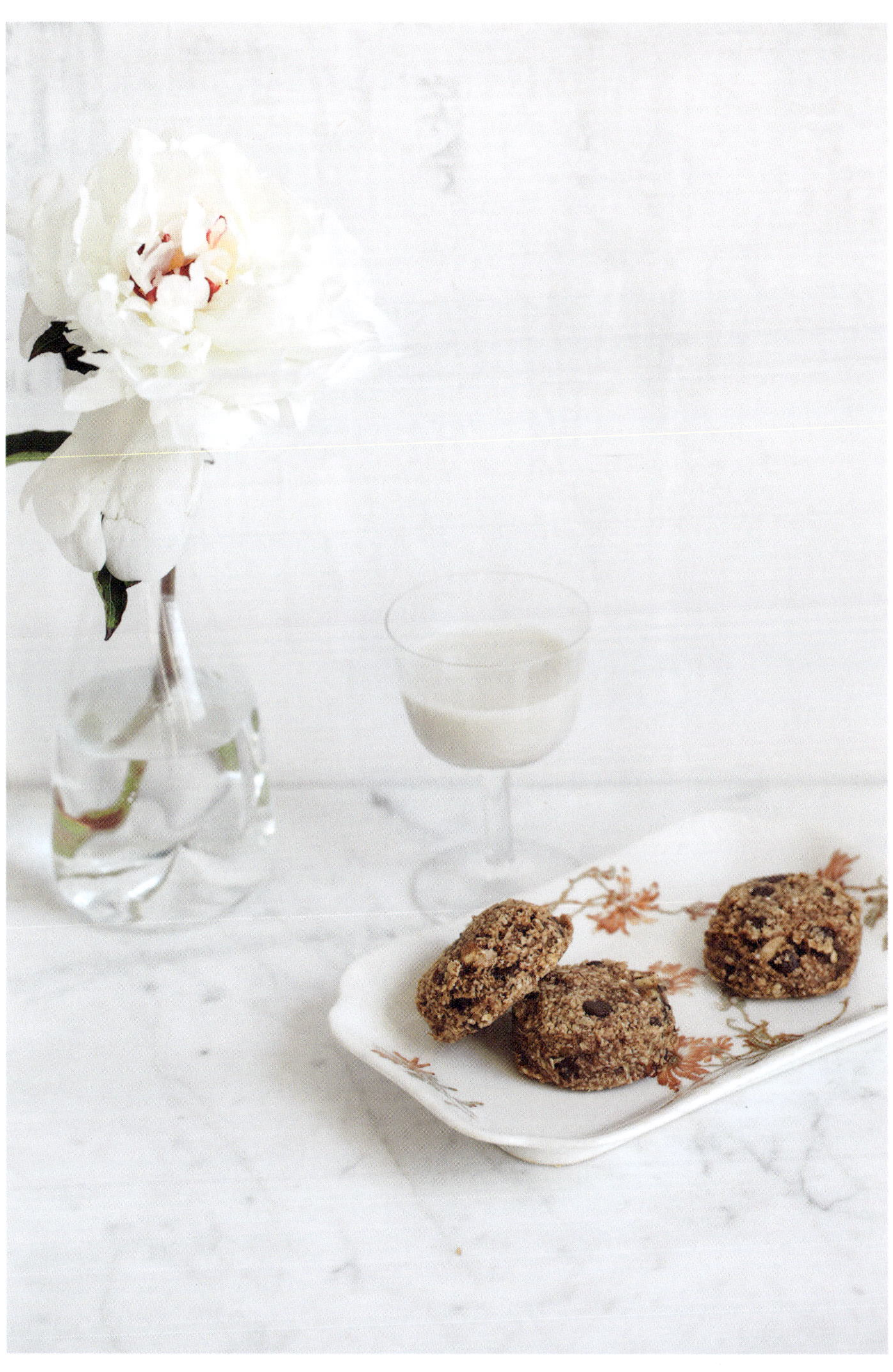

Cocoa Cupcakes

These cupcakes are one of the first recipes I ever made. I managed to convince my dad they weren't vegan and gluten-free (even though they totally are!), and they have been enjoyed by Anthony Bourdain, who was famously anti-vegan and anti-dessert.

YIELD: 12 cupcakes

CUPCAKES
2 cups (480 ml) unsweetened chocolate almond milk
2 teaspoons apple cider vinegar
2 cups (296 g) gluten-free 1-to-1 flour
¾ cup (65 g) unsweetened cocoa powder
½ cup (77 g) date sugar (or maple sugar)
2 teaspoons baking powder
2 teaspoons baking soda
1 teaspoon salt
½ teaspoon ground cinnamon
½ teaspoon pumpkin pie spice (for homemade pumpkin pie spice, mix ½ teaspoon ground cinnamon, ⅛ teaspoon ground cloves, ¼ teaspoon ground ginger, and ⅛ teaspoon ground nutmeg)
½ cup (100 g) melted raw extra-virgin coconut oil
½ cup (120 ml) maple syrup
½ cup (122 g) unsweetened applesauce
1 tablespoon (15 ml) vanilla extract
1 teaspoon almond extract (optional)

ICING
½ cup (128 g) sweet potato purée
¼ cup (64 g) cashew butter
¼ cup (30 g) carob powder
3 tablespoons (29 g) date sugar
4 ounces (112 g) vegan sugar-free chocolate chips
2 tablespoons (28 g) raw extra-virgin coconut oil
10 to 15 drops vanilla stevia
Pinch of salt

Sending Love Meditation

You're the one who truly suffers by holding a grudge. The antidote to this darkness is to turn on the lights, so flip on the switch in the heavy room of your heart. I promise you will start to feel that weight lift.

Sit cross-legged with your palms facing up and eyes closed. Take long, deep breaths and visualize the person you find difficult sitting in front of you. Take a deep breath in and send that person a stream of love from your heart center. Allow this love to look like whatever comes up for you (a ray of red light, a bright white stream of energy, etc.). See it on your exhale going straight into their heart center. On your inhale, envision yourself receiving love back from their heart center and repeat. After a minute or so, the two of you should be surrounded with light and love, in a bubble of your mutual energies. Take a deep breath in and hold this light and love. Bow your head to this person and silently say a little prayer or wish for their well-being. Exhale and relax. Continue this meditation for at least 40 days.

Preheat the oven to 375°F (190°C, or gas mark 5) and line a 12-cup muffin pan with paper baking cups.

To make the cupcakes, combine the chocolate almond milk and apple cider vinegar in a large measuring cup, stir, and set aside to curdle.

Meanwhile, combine all the dry ingredients together in a stand mixer or medium mixing bowl and mix well until the mixture is clump-free.

Pour in the coconut oil, maple syrup, applesauce, and extracts. Add the curdled chocolate almond milk and mix at medium-low speed (or by hand) until the ingredients are thoroughly combined. Using an ice-cream scooper or tablespoon, fill each cup three-quarters of the way with batter. Bake for 15 to 17 minutes, or until a toothpick inserted into the center of a cupcake comes out clean. Set aside to cool.

To make the icing, combine the sweet potato purée, cashew butter, carob powder, and date sugar in a stand mixer, blender, or food processor and mix. Set aside.

Fill a medium saucepan halfway with water and bring to a boil. Place the chocolate chips and coconut oil in a separate smaller saucepan, place pan in the hot water, and heat, stirring continuously for 3 to 5 minutes, or until most of the chocolate has melted. Pour the chocolate into a mixing bowl with the mixture from step 5, add the vanilla stevia and salt, and mix thoroughly. Put the bowl in the refrigerator and chill for 30 to 60 minutes.

Mix the icing on high speed for a few minutes until thick and creamy. Ice the cupcakes immediately and serve!

“

I send love to those whom I find most difficult.

Vanilla Chai Cupcakes

When I first started selling my cupcakes at small fairs and pop-up shops, I didn't offer vanilla because I had more creative flavors. But kids would always want vanilla! So, I went into the kitchen and made these cupcakes for the kiddos with all the love in my heart. Anchoring yourself in the pureness of your true intentions will shine in every area of your life.

YIELD: 12 cupcakes

CUPCAKES

2 cups (480 ml) unsweetened vanilla almond milk
2 teaspoons apple cider vinegar
2 chai tea bags
2 cups (224 g) quinoa flour
½ cup (77 g) date sugar
2 teaspoons baking powder
2 teaspoons baking soda
1 teaspoon ground cinnamon
1 teaspoon ground nutmeg
1 teaspoon ground cloves
1 teaspoon salt
½ cup (100 g) melted raw extra-virgin coconut oil
½ cup (120 ml) maple syrup
½ cup (122 g) unsweetened applesauce
1 tablespoon (15 ml) vanilla extract
1 teaspoon almond extract
1 cup (86 g) unsweetened coconut flakes, for decorating

ICING

1 cup (192 g) nonhydrogenated shortening
¼ cup (60 ml) coconut cream
¼ cup (60 ml) maple syrup or brown-rice syrup
3 tablespoons (48 g) cashew butter
1 teaspoon ground nutmeg
1 teaspoon ground cloves
1 teaspoon vanilla extract
2 teaspoons almond extract
1 teaspoon ground cinnamon

SPICE BLEND

½ teaspoon ground cinnamon
½ teaspoon ground nutmeg
½ teaspoon ground cloves

“

My pure intentions radiate outward.

Preheat the oven to 375°F (190°C, or gas mark 5) and line a 12-cup muffin pan with paper baking cups.

To make the cupcakes, combine the almond milk and apple cider vinegar in a large measuring cup, stir, and then add the tea bags. Set it aside to steep (the mixture should curdle).

Meanwhile, combine all the dry ingredients together in a stand mixer or medium mixing bowl and mix well until clump-free. Add the coconut oil, maple syrup, applesauce, and extracts.

Remove the tea bags from the measuring cup and pour the curdled tea into the batter. Mix at medium-low speed (or by hand) until the ingredients are thoroughly combined. Using an ice-cream scooper or tablespoon, fill each cup three-quarters of the way with batter. Bake for 15 to 17 minutes, or until a toothpick inserted into the center of a cupcake comes out clean. Set aside to cool.

Meanwhile, make the icing. Combine all the ingredients in a bowl and whip at medium-high speed until fluffy and creamy. Ice the cupcakes and top with coconut flakes.

Combine the spice blend ingredients and sprinkle over the cupcakes.

A Meditation to Purify Intentions

Sit comfortably with your eyes closed and your palms facing up. Take a few long, deep breaths and center yourself in the quiet within you. Bring to mind a troubled area of your life. Look at the intention that's currently behind the wheel. See it clearly, without any judgment. Now bring up these questions: What do I truly desire? How do I really want to operate in this area? Let your true intentions float to the surface and then sit in what should feel like a shift in your being. When you are ready, take a deep breath in, holding it and letting it soak into every cell of your being. Exhale.

CONCLUSION
Dear Sweet Reader

You made it!

And yet, you are only at the beginning of this glorious lifelong journey to love and honor your body, to navigate this wondrous world with your inner compass. Take all the tools you have learned here and keep them in your back pocket. Take the nuggets of wisdom that appeal to you and keep those close to your heart. Let yourself be a constant work in progress so the pitfalls don't paralyze you. Jump back on the horse and keep riding.

It's been an honor to guide you through this book, and if you need further support, it doesn't have to end here. Head over to *www.CassandraBodzak.com/themindfultable* for many free resources—meditations, cooking videos, and advice—to enrich your own journey to eat with intention. I've also got a special bonus chapter to take you behind the scenes of my postpartum journey.

Spoiler alert: I had to go back and re-learn all the concepts I teach in this book as I struggled to re-heal my relationship with my body after having my son. Say hi to me on social media at @CassandraBodzak, watch me on YouTube at @CassandraBodzakTV, or get my free weekly newsletter at cassandrabodzak.substack.com. I would LOVE to hear from you and see your food photos and your #MindfulTable book #shelfies. Show me where you are bringing this book, what meditations you love, and what really hit home for you along your journey. I'll say hi right back and share it with the rest of our amazing community!

May you always eat with intention and live a life that LIGHTS you up,

Cassandra

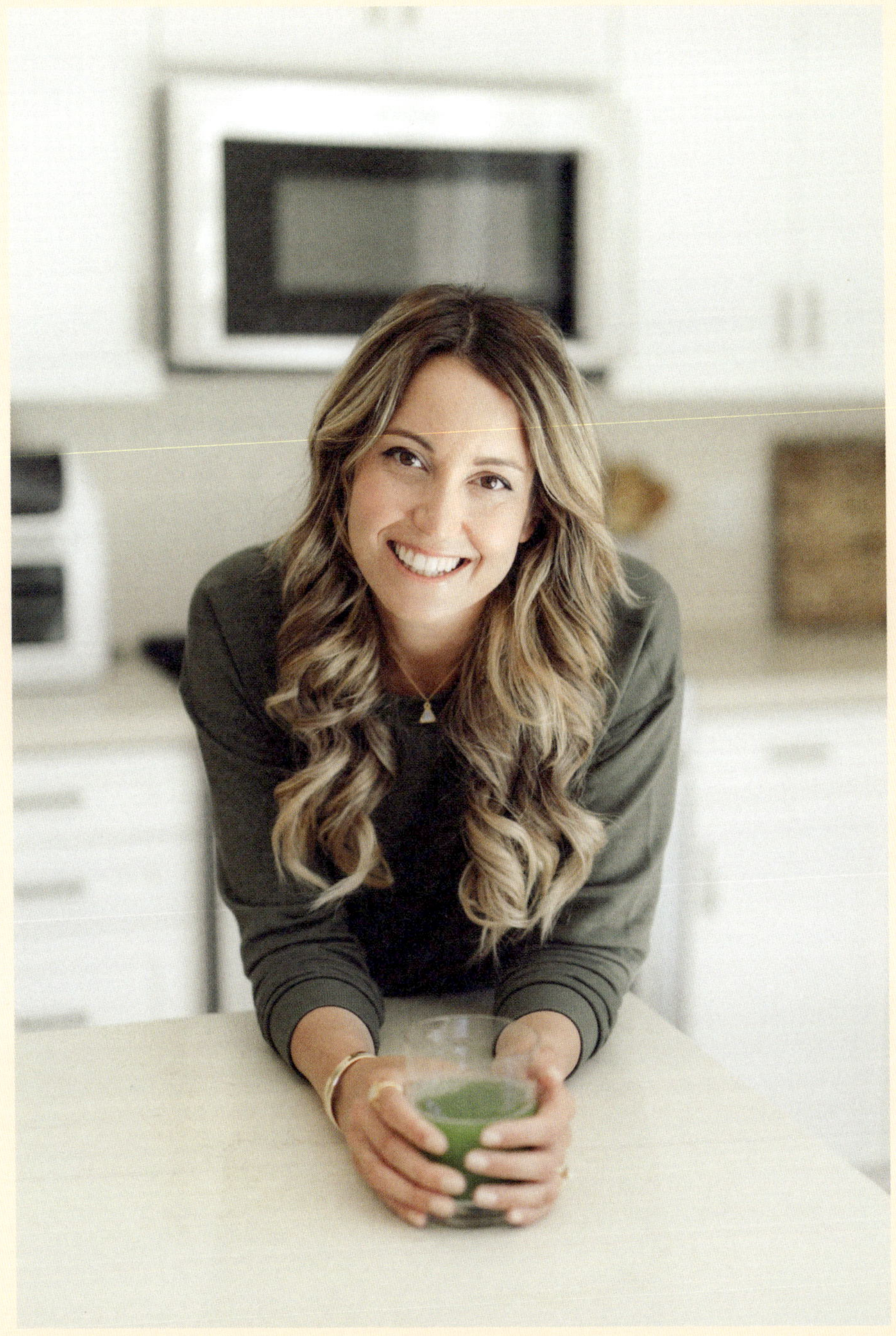

Index

ACKNOWLEDGMENTS

I would like to thank Jeannine Dillon and the entire Quarto family for taking a risk on something that was unlike any cookbook or lifestyle manual out there—for having faith in my vision of a world where people love and listen to their bodies, and ultimately have a deeper connection with their soul.

I would like to thank Rage Kindelsperger for recognizing that this book was ahead of its time and breathing new life into it now.

I'm so grateful to the wonderful Natalie Butterfield for your patience, grace, and expertise while editing this book to fit its new size. Thank you for making me feel seen and heard every step of the way.

Thank you to the wonderful Quarto design team for being so kind and collaborative. You made this book exquisitely gorgeous.

I would like to thank Rossella Rago, the Veronica to my Betty in the kitchen and one of my dearest friends, for passing along a note that I might be a great fit for a juice book, and for all the magic that ensued following that little flap of a butterfly's wings. This book wouldn't exist without your love and support, and I'm eternally grateful.

I would like to thank Mary Aracena, for being the best assistant, friend, recipe helper, and all-around support system during the creation of this book. I know I will fondly look back on those twelve-hour days we spent together laughing, crying, eating lots of food, and having minor breakdowns in the kitchen for the rest of my life. Your beautiful energy is infused in every corner of this book. You are truly a living angel and I am incredibly grateful to have had you by my side during this magical time.

I would like to thank my parents, Ken and Debbie Bodzak, for having infinite amounts of patience with my always needing to take the road less traveled and often dancing to the beat of my own drummer. I am sure it hasnt been the easiest having me as a daughter, and you both have been so loving, supportive, and encouraging through it all. Thank you for cheering me on. Love you both tons. "Look, guys, I finally wrote the book!!" :)

Lastly, I would like to thank my grandma, Joan McDonald, for always being a steady rock in my life, an open ear, and a wise advisor. Your grace and courage in this life inspires me to constantly be a better version of myself, your patience and faith remind me to not sweat the small stuff (and its all small stuff), and your love always feels like a bright ray of sunshine on my day. Love you madly.

I dedicate this book to my brother, Kenneth Bodzak, whose health journey inspired me to start sharing my own recipes and discoveries.

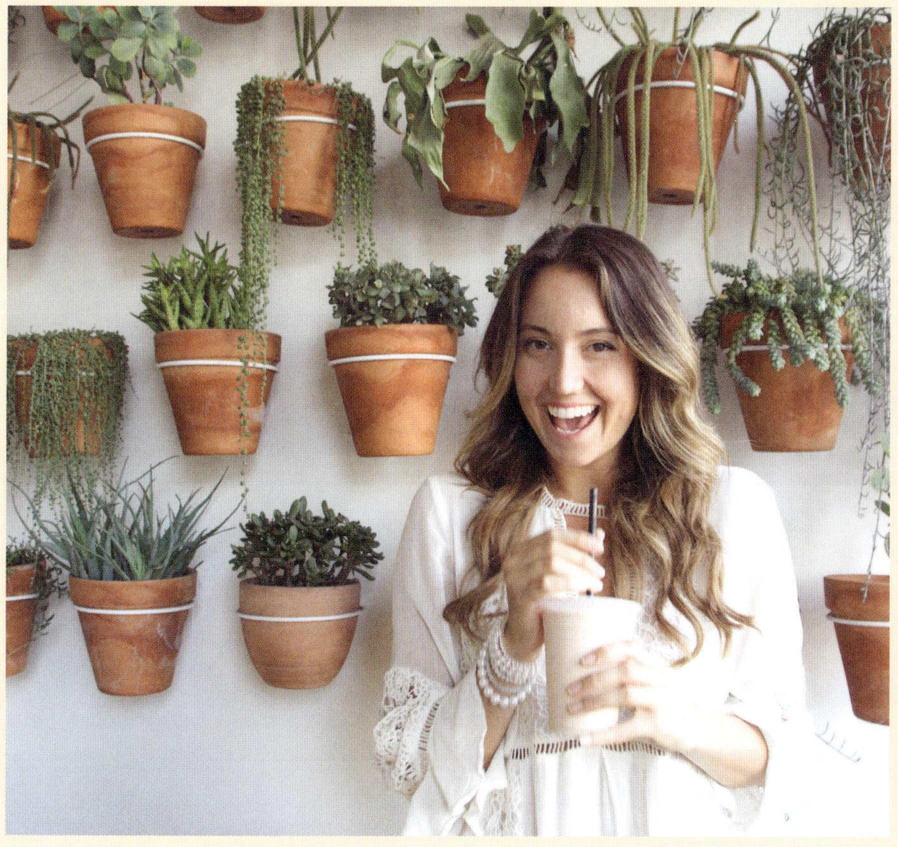

ABOUT THE AUTHOR

CASSANDRA BODZAK is an actress, best-selling author, and certified holistic health and lifestyle coach. She studied health, wellness, and lifestyle coaching at Harvard Medical School. She also hosts the podcast *You with Intention*, and creates free food, meditation, and intentional living content on her YouTube channel, *CassandraBodzakTV*.

Cassandra helps women all over the world get back into alignment with their soul, nourish themselves both physically and spiritually, and consciously create the life they desire.

You may have seen Cassandra on ABC's *The Taste* with Anthony Bourdain as the "happy, healthy living guru." She has also been named "an award-winning thought leader and intuitive coach" by Forbes and "a spiritual leader" by *Well + Good*.

This edition published in 2026 by Rock Point,
an imprint of The Quarto Group,
142 West 36th Street, 4th Floor,
New York, NY 10018, USA
(212) 779-4972
www.Quarto.com

First published in 2016 as *Eat with Intention* by Race Point Publishing, an imprint of the Quarto Group, 142 West 36th Street, 4th Floor, New York, NY 10018, USA.

EEA Representation, WTS Tax d.o.o.,
Žanova ulica 3, 4000 Kranj, Slovenia.
www.wts-tax.si

Rock Point titles are also available at discount for retail, wholesale, promotional, and bulk purchase. For details, contact the Special Sales Manager by email at specialsales@quarto.com or by mail at The Quarto Group, Attn: Special Sales Manager, 100 Cummings Center Suite 265D, Beverly, MA 01915 USA.

10 9 8 7 6 5 4 3 2 1

ISBN: 978-1-57715-690-1

Digital edition published in 2026
eISBN: 978-1-57715-691-8

Library of Congress Cataloging-in-Publication Data available upon request.

Publisher: Rage Kindelsperger
Creative Director: Laura Drew
Managing Editor: Cara Donaldson
Editor: Natalie Butterfield
Photography: Evi Abeler, except where noted; Unsplash: 2 (Christine), 4 (Glen-Carrie) 16 (Priscilla du Preez), 29 (feey), 63 (Melody Zimmerman); 18 (Cassandra Bodzak); 19, 159 (Kaysha Weiner); Alamy: 36 (The Picture Pantry Ltd); Freepik: 93, 127; Getty: 125 (Anne DEL SOCORRO); 167 (Danielle Jenkens); Shutterstock: 18, 53, 69, 91, 99, 102, 111, 117, 125, 144, 147
Shoot Assistant: Harriet Honkaniemi
Food Stylist: Mariana Velasquez
Assistant Food Stylists: Kristin Stangl and Erika Joyce
Cover and Interior Design: Vanessa Masci

Printed in Huizhou, Guangdong, China TT102025